Underground Clinical Vignettes

Microbiology I: Immunology, Parasitology, Urology, and Mycology

FIFTH EDITION

D1254024

Underground Clinical Vignettes

Microbiology I: Immunology, Parasitology, Urology, and Mycology

FIFTH EDITION

Todd A. Swanson, M.D., Ph.D.
Resident in Radiation Oncology
William Beaumont Hospital
Royal Oak, Michigan

Sandra I. Kim, M.D., Ph.D.
Resident in Internal Medicine
Beth Israel Deaconess Medical Center
Harvard Medical School
Boston, Massachusetts

Olga E. Flomin, M.D.
Resident in Obstetrics and Gynecology
William Beaumont Hospital
Royal Oak, Michigan

⊕. Wolters Kluwer | Lippincott Williams & Wilkins
Health

Philadelphia • Baltimore • New York • London
Buenos Aires • Hong Kong • Sydney • Tokyo

Acquisitions Editor: Nancy Anastasi Duffy
Developmental Editor: Kathleen H. Scogna
Managing Editor: Nancy Hoffmann
Marketing Manager: Jennifer Kuklinski
Associate Production Manager: Kevin P. Johnson
Creative Director: Doug Smock
Compositor: International Typesetting and Composition
Printer: R.R. Donnelley & Son's—Crawfordsville

Copyright © 2008 Lippincott Williams & Wilkins, a Wolters Kluwer business

351 West Camden Street
Baltimore, MD 21201

530 Walnut Street
Philadelphia, PA 19106

All rights reserved. This book is protected by copyright. No part of this book may be reproduced in any form or by any means, including photocopying, or utilized by any information storage and retrieval system without written permission from the copyright owner.

The publisher is not responsible (as a matter of product liability, negligence, or otherwise) for any injury resulting from any material contained herein. This publication contains information relating to general principles of medical care that should not be construed as specific instructions for individual patients. Manufacturers' product information and package inserts should be reviewed for current information, including contraindications, dosages, and precautions.

Printed in the United States of America

First Edition, 2001 Blackwell Publishing Inc.
Second Edition, 2003 Blackwell Publishing Inc.
Third Edition, 2005 Blackwell Publishing Inc.
Fourth Edition, 2005 Blackwell Publishing Inc.

Library of Congress Cataloging-in-Publication Data

Swanson, Todd A.
   Microbiology / Todd Swanson, Sandra Kim, Olga E. Flomin.—5th ed.
       p. ; cm.—(Underground clinical vignettes)
   Rev. ed. of: Microbiology / Vikas Bhushan . . . [et al.]. 4th ed. c2005.
   Includes bibliographical references and index.
   ISBN-13: 978-0-7817-6471-1 (alk. paper)
   ISBN-10: 0-7817-6471-8 (alk. paper)
   1. Medical microbiology—Case studies.   2. Physicians—Licenses—United
States—Examinations—Study guides.   I. Kim, Sandra.   II. Flomin, Olga E.
III. Microbiology.   IV. Title.   V. Series.
   [DNLM: 1. Microbiology—Case Reports.   2. Microbiology—Problems
and Exercises.   QW 18.2 S972m 2007]
   QR46.B465 2007
   616.9'041—dc22

                                                            2007003561

The publishers have made every effort to trace the copyright holders for borrowed material. If they have inadvertently overlooked any, they will be pleased to make the necessary arrangements at the first opportunity.

To purchase additional copies of this book, call our customer service department at **(800) 638-3030** or fax orders to **(301) 223-2320**. International customers should call **(301) 223-2300**.

Visit Lippincott Williams & Wilkins on the Internet: http://www.LWW.com. Lippincott Williams & Wilkins customer service representatives are available from 8:30 am to 6:00 pm, EST.

07 08 09 10
1 2 3 4 5 6 7 8 9 10

dedications

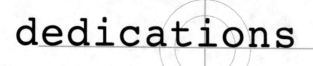

For Natan and Marina,
for whose encouragement and assistance we are eternally grateful.

preface

First published in 1999, the Underground Clinical Vignettes series has provided thousands of students with a highly effective review tool as they prepare for medical exams, particularly the USMLE Step 1 and 2 exams. Designed as a quick study guide, each UCV book contains patient-centered clinical cases that highlight a range of medical diagnoses.

With this new edition of Underground Clinical Vignettes, we have incorporated feedback from medical students across the country to provide updated cases with expanded treatment and discussion sections. A new two-page format enables readers to formulate an initial diagnosis prior to reading the answer, while the added differential diagnosis section encourages critical thinking about comparable cases. The inclusion of relevant magnetic resonance images, radiographs, and photographs allows students to visualize the physical presentation of each case more readily. Breakout points, tables, and algorithms have been added, along with all new board-format questions-and-answers, making this edition of UCV an ideal source of information for exam review, classroom discussion, or clinical rotations.

The clinical vignettes in this series are designed to give added emphasis to pathogenesis, epidemiology, management, and complications. Although each case tends to present all the signs, symptoms, and diagnostic findings for a particular illness, patients generally will not present with such a "complete" picture either clinically or on a medical examination. Cases are not meant to simulate a potential real patient or an examination vignette.

Access to the LWW online companion site, ThePoint, will be offered as a premium with the purchase of the Underground Clinical Vignettes Step 1 bundle. Benefits include an online test link and additional new board-format questions covering all UCV subject areas.

We hope you will find the Underground Clinical Vignettes series informative and useful. We welcome any feedback, suggestions, or corrections you have about this series. Please contact us at LWW.com/medstudent.

contributors

Series Editors

Todd A. Swanson, M.D., Ph.D.
Resident in Radiation Oncology
William Beaumont Hospital
Royal Oak, Michigan

Sandra I. Kim, M.D., Ph.D.
Resident in Internal Medicine
Beth Israel Deaconess Medical Center
Harvard Medical School
Boston, Massachusetts

Series Contributors

Olga E. Flomin, M.D.
Resident in Obstetrics and Gynecology
William Beaumont Hospital
Royal Oak, Michigan

Medina C. Kushen, M.D.
Resident in Neurosurgery
University of Chicago Hospitals
Chicago, Illinois

Marc J. Glucksman, Ph.D.
Professor of Biochemistry and Molecular Biology
Director, Midwest Proteome Center and
Co-Director, Rosalind Franklin Structural Biology Laboratories
Rosalind Franklin University of Medicine and Science
The Chicago Medical School
North Chicago, Illinois

acknowledgments

Thanks to Dr. Alvaro Martinez, Dr. Larry Kestin, and the entire radiation oncology program at William Beaumont Hospital for allowing the flexibility to work on this project during an already vigorous residency training program.

— Todd A. Swanson

Thanks to Todd for his work on this series.

— Sandra I. Kim

abbreviations

ABGs	arterial blood gases	BPH	benign prostatic hypertrophy
ABPA	allergic bronchopulmonary aspergillosis	BUN	blood urea nitrogen
		CABG	coronary artery bypass grafting
ACA	anticardiolipin antibody	CAD	coronary artery disease
ACE	angiotensin-converting enzyme	CaEDTA	calcium edetate
ACL	anterior cruciate ligament	CALLA	common acute lymphoblastic leukemia antigen
ACTH	adrenocorticotropic hormone		
AD	adjustment disorder	cAMP	cyclic adenosine monophosphate
ADA	adenosine deaminase		
ADD	attention deficit disorder	C-ANCA	cytoplasmic antineutrophil cytoplasmic antibody
ADH	antidiuretic hormone		
ADHD	attention deficit hyperactivity disorder	CBC	complete blood count
		CBD	common bile duct
ADP	adenosine diphosphate	CCU	cardiac care unit
AFO	ankle-foot orthosis	CD	cluster of differentiation
AFP	α-fetoprotein	2-CdA	2-chlorodeoxyadenosine
AIDS	acquired immunodeficiency syndrome	CEA	carcinoembryonic antigen
		CFTR	cystic fibrosis transmembrane conductance regulator
ALL	acute lymphocytic leukemia		
ALS	amyotrophic lateral sclerosis	cGMP	cyclic guanosine monophosphate
ALT	alanine aminotransferase		
AML	acute myelogenous leukemia	CHF	congestive heart failure
ANA	antinuclear antibody	CK	creatine kinase
Angio	angiography	CK-MB	creatine kinase, MB fraction
AP	anteroposterior	CLL	chronic lymphocytic leukemia
APKD	adult polycystic kidney disease	CML	chronic myelogenous leukemia
aPTT	activated partial thromboplastin time	CMV	cytomegalovirus
		CN	cranial nerve
ARDS	adult respiratory distress syndrome	CNS	central nervous system
		COPD	chronic obstructive pulmonary disease
5-ASA	5-aminosalicylic acid		
ASCA	antibodies to *Saccharomyces cerevisiae*	COX	cyclooxygenase
		CP	cerebellopontine
ASO	antistreptolysin O	CPAP	continuous positive airway pressure
AST	aspartate aminotransferase		
ATLL	adult T-cell leukemia/lymphoma	CPK	creatine phosphokinase
ATPase	adenosine triphosphatase	CPPD	calcium pyrophosphate dihydrate
AV	arteriovenous, atrioventricular		
AZT	azidothymidine (zidovudine)	CPR	cardiopulmonary resuscitation
BAL	British antilewisite (dimercaprol)	CREST	calcinosis, Raynaud phenomenon, esophageal involvement, sclerodactyly, telangiectasia (syndrome)
BCG	bacille Calmette-Guérin		
BE	barium enema		
b.i.d.	twice a day		
BP	blood pressure	CRP	C-reactive protein

CSF	cerebrospinal fluid
CSOM	chronic suppurative otitis media
CT	cardiac transplant, computed tomography
CVA	cerebrovascular accident
CXR	chest x-ray
d4T	didehydrodeoxythymidine (stavudine)
DCS	decompression sickness
DDH	developmental dysplasia of the hip
ddI	dideoxyinosine (didanosine)
DES	diethylstilbestrol
DEXA	dual-energy x-ray absorptiometry
DHEAS	dehydroepiandrosterone sulfate
DIC	disseminated intravascular coagulation
DIF	direct immunofluorescence
DIP	distal interphalangeal (joint)
DKA	diabetic ketoacidosis
DL_{co}	diffusing capacity of carbon monoxide
DMSA	2,3-dimercaptosuccinic acid
DNA	deoxyribonucleic acid
DNase	deoxyribonuclease
2,3-DPG	2,3-diphosphoglycerate
dsDNA	double-stranded DNA
DSM	Diagnostic and Statistical Manual
dsRNA	double-stranded RNA
DTP	diphtheria, tetanus, pertussis (vaccine)
DTPA	diethylenetriamine-penta-acetic acid
DTs	delirium tremens
DVT	deep venous thrombosis
EBV	Epstein-Barr virus
ECG	electrocardiography
Echo	echocardiography
ECM	erythema chronicum migrans
ECT	electroconvulsive therapy
EEG	electroencephalography
EF	ejection fraction, elongation factor
EGD	esophagogastroduodenoscopy
EHEC	enterohemorrhagic *E. coli*
EIA	enzyme immunoassay
ELISA	enzyme-linked immunosorbent assay

EM	electron microscopy
EMG	electromyography
ENT	ears, nose, and throat
EPVE	early prosthetic valve endocarditis
ER	emergency room
ERCP	endoscopic retrograde cholangiopancreatography
ERT	estrogen replacement therapy
ESR	erythrocyte sedimentation rate
ETEC	enterotoxigenic *E. coli*
EtOH	ethanol
FAP	familial adenomatous polyposis
FEV_1	forced expiratory volume in 1 second
FH	familial hypercholesterolemia
FNA	fine-needle aspiration
FSH	follicle-stimulating hormone
FTA-ABS	fluorescent treponemal antibody absorption test
FVC	forced vital capacity
G6PD	glucose-6-phosphate dehydrogenase
GABA	gamma-aminobutyric acid
GERD	gastroesophageal reflux disease
GFR	glomerular filtration rate
GGT	gamma-glutamyltransferase
GH	growth hormone
GI	gastrointestinal
GnRH	gonadotropin-releasing hormone
GU	genitourinary
GVHD	graft-versus-host disease
HAART	highly active antiretroviral therapy
HAV	hepatitis A virus
Hb	hemoglobin
HbA-1C	hemoglobin A-1C
HBsAg	hepatitis B surface antigen
HBV	hepatitis B virus
hCG	human chorionic gonadotropin
HCO_3	bicarbonate
Hct	hematocrit
HCV	hepatitis C virus
HDL	high-density lipoprotein
HDL-C	high-density lipoprotein-cholesterol
HEENT	head, eyes, ears, nose, and throat (exam)
HELLP	hemolysis, elevated LFTs, low platelets (syndrome)

HFMD	hand, foot, and mouth disease	LDL	low-density lipoprotein
HGPRT	hypoxanthine-guanine phosphoribosyltransferase	LE	lupus erythematosus (cell)
		LES	lower esophageal sphincter
5-HIAA	5-hydroxindoleacetic acid	LFTs	liver function tests
HIDA	hepato-iminodiacetic acid (scan)	LH	luteinizing hormone
HIV	human immunodeficiency virus	LMN	lower motor neuron
HLA	human leukocyte antigen	LP	lumbar puncture
HMG-CoA	hydroxymethylglutaryl-coenzyme A	LPVE	late prosthetic valve endocarditis
		L/S	lecithin-sphingomyelin (ratio)
HMP	hexose monophosphate	LSD	lysergic acid diethylamide
HPI	history of present illness	LT	labile toxin
HPV	human papillomavirus	LV	left ventricular
HR	heart rate	LVH	left ventricular hypertrophy
HRIG	human rabies immune globulin	Lytes	electrolytes
HRS	hepatorenal syndrome	Mammo	mammography
HRT	hormone replacement therapy	MAO	monoamine oxidase (inhibitor)
HSG	hysterosalpingography	MCP	metacarpophalangeal (joint)
HSV	herpes simplex virus	MCTD	mixed connective tissue disorder
HTLV	human T-cell leukemia virus	MCV	mean corpuscular volume
HUS	hemolytic-uremic syndrome	MEN	multiple endocrine neoplasia
HVA	homovanillic acid	MI	myocardial infarction
ICP	intracranial pressure	MIBG	meta-iodobenzylguanidine (radioisotope)
ICU	intensive care unit		
ID/CC	identification and chief complaint	MMR	measles, mumps, rubella (vaccine)
IDDM	insulin dependent diabetes mellitus		
		MPGN	membranoproliferative glomerulonephritis
IFA	immunofluorescent antibody		
Ig	immunoglobulin	MPS	mucopolysaccharide
IGF	insulin like growth factor	MPTP	1-methyl-4-phenyl-tetrahydropyridine
IHSS	idiopathic hypertrophic subaortic stenosis		
		MR	magnetic resonance (imaging)
IM	intramuscular	mRNA	messenger ribonucleic acid
IMA	inferior mesenteric artery	MRSA	methicillin-resistant *S. aureus*
INH	isoniazid	MTP	metatarsophalangeal (joint)
INR	International Normalized Ratio	NAD	nicotinamide adenine dinucleotide
IP_3	inositol 1,4,5-triphosphate		
IPF	idiopathic pulmonary fibrosis	NADP	nicotinamide adenine dinucleotide phosphate
ITP	idiopathic thrombocytopenic purpura		
		NADPH	reduced nicotinamide adenine dinucleotide phosphate
IUD	intrauterine device		
IV	intravenous	NF	neurofibromatosis
IVC	inferior vena cava	NIDDM	non–insulin-dependent diabetes mellitus
IVIG	intravenous immunoglobulin		
IVP	intravenous pyelography	NNRTI	non-nucleoside reverse transcriptase inhibitor
JRA	juvenile rheumatoid arthritis		
JVP	jugular venous pressure	NO	nitric oxide
KOH	potassium hydroxide	NPO	nil per os (nothing by mouth)
KUB	kidney, ureter, bladder	NSAID	nonsteroidal anti-inflammatory drug
LCM	lymphocytic choriomeningitis		
LDH	lactate dehydrogenase	Nuc	nuclear medicine

NYHA	New York Heart Association	PROM	premature rupture of membranes
OB	obstetric	PSA	prostate-specific antigen
OCD	obsessive-compulsive disorder	PSS	progressive systemic sclerosis
OCPs	oral contraceptive pills	PT	prothrombin time
OR	operating room	PTH	parathyroid hormone
PA	posteroanterior	PTSD	post-traumatic stress disorder
PABA	para-aminobenzoic acid	PTT	partial thromboplastin time
PAN	polyarteritis nodosa	PUVA	psoralen ultraviolet A
P-ANCA	perinuclear antineutrophil cytoplasmic antibody	PVC	premature ventricular contraction
Pao_2	partial pressure of oxygen in arterial blood	q.i.d.	four times a day
		RA	rheumatoid arthritis
PAS	periodic acid Schiff	RAIU	radioactive iodine uptake
PAT	paroxysmal atrial tachycardia	RAST	radioallergosorbent test
PBS	peripheral blood smear	RBC	red blood cell
Pco_2	partial pressure of carbon dioxide	REM	rapid eye movement
		RES	reticuloendothelial system
PCOM	posterior communicating (artery)	RFFIT	rapid fluorescent focus inhibition test
PCOS	polycystic ovarian syndrome	RFTs	renal function tests
PCP	phencyclidine	RHD	rheumatic heart disease
PCR	polymerase chain reaction	RNA	ribonucleic acid
PCT	porphyria cutanea tarda	RNP	ribonucleoprotein
PCTA	percutaneous coronary transluminal angioplasty	RPR	rapid plasma reagin
		RR	respiratory rate
PCV	polycythemia vera	RSV	respiratory syncytial virus
PDA	patent ductus arteriosus	RUQ	right upper quadrant
PDGF	platelet-derived growth factor	RV	residual volume
PE	physical exam	Sao_2	oxygen saturation in arterial blood
PEFR	peak expiratory flow rate		
PEG	polyethylene glycol	SBFT	small bowel follow-through
PEPCK	phosphoenolpyruvate carboxykinase	SCC	squamous cell carcinoma
		SCID	severe combined immunodeficiency
PET	positron emission tomography		
PFTs	pulmonary function tests	SERM	selective estrogen receptor modulator
PID	pelvic inflammatory disease		
PIP	proximal interphalangeal (joint)	SGOT	serum glutamic-oxaloacetic transaminase
PKU	phenylketonuria		
PMDD	premenstrual dysphoric disorder	SIADH	syndrome of inappropriate antidiuretic hormone
PML	progressive multifocal leukoencephalopathy		
		SIDS	sudden infant death syndrome
PMN	polymorphonuclear (leukocyte)	SLE	systemic lupus erythematosus
PNET	primitive neuroectodermal tumor	SMA	superior mesenteric artery
PNH	paroxysmal nocturnal hemoglobinuria	SSPE	subacute sclerosing panencephalitis
Po_2	partial pressure of oxygen	SSRI	selective serotonin reuptake inhibitor
PPD	purified protein derivative (of tuberculosis)		
		ST	stable toxin
PPH	primary postpartum hemorrhage	STD	sexually transmitted disease
PRA	panel reactive antibody		

T2W	T2-weighted (MRI)	TXA	thromboxane A
T_3	triiodothyronine	UA	urinalysis
T_4	thyroxine	UDCA	ursodeoxycholic acid
TAH-BSO	total abdominal hysterectomy–bilateral salpingo-oophorectomy	UGI	upper GI
		UPPP	uvulopalatopharyngoplasty
TB	tuberculosis	URI	upper respiratory infection
TCA	tricyclic antidepressant	US	ultrasound
TCC	transitional cell carcinoma	UTI	urinary tract infection
TDT	terminal deoxytransferase	UV	ultraviolet
TFTs	thyroid function tests	VDRL	Venereal Disease Research Laboratory
TGF	transforming growth factor		
THC	tetrahydrocannabinol	VIN	vulvar intraepithelial neoplasia
TIA	transient ischemic attack	VIP	vasoactive intestinal polypeptide
t.i.d.	three times a day	VLDL	very low density lipoprotein
TIPS	transjugular intrahepatic portosystemic shunt	VMA	vanillylmandelic acid
		V/Q	ventilation/perfusion (ratio)
TLC	total lung capacity	VRE	vancomycin-resistant enterococcus
TMP-SMX	trimethoprim-sulfamethoxazole		
tPA	tissue plasminogen activator	VS	vital signs
TP-HA	*Treponema pallidum* hemagglutination assay	VSD	ventricular septal defect
		vWF	von Willebrand factor
TPP	thiamine pyrophosphate	VZV	varicella-zoster virus
TRAP	tartrate-resistant acid phosphatase	WAGR	Wilms tumor, aniridia, genitourinary abnormalities, mental retardation (syndrome)
tRNA	transfer ribonucleic acid		
TSH	thyroid-stimulating hormone	WBC	white blood cell
TSS	toxic shock syndrome	WHI	Women's Health Initiative
TTP	thrombotic thrombocytopenic purpura	WPW	Wolff-Parkinson-White syndrome
TURP	transurethral resection of the prostate	XR	x-ray
		ZN	Ziehl-Neelsen (stain)

Underground Clinical Vignettes

Vignettes

Microbiology I: Immunology, Parasitology, Urology, and Mycology

FIFTH EDITION

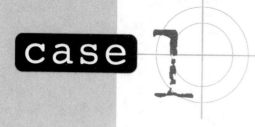

ID/CC	A 17-year-old boy presents with **itchy eyes**, nasal stuffiness, increased lacrimation, **sneezing**, and a **watery nasal discharge**.
HPI	He has had similar episodes in the past that have corresponded with **changing of the seasons**. His mother is known to have bronchial asthma.
PE	VS: no fever. PE: pallor; **boggy nasal mucosa; nasal polyps present;** conjunctiva congested; no exudate.
Labs	Conjunctival and nasal smear demonstrates presence of **eosinophils**; no bacteria on Gram stain; no neutrophils. Allergen skin tests (sensitized cutaneous mast cells) show positive sensitivity.
Gross Pathology	Nasal mucosa hyperemic and swollen with fluid transudation.

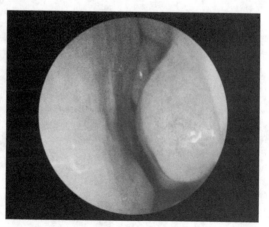

Figure 1-1. Swollen left inferior turbinate.

Micro Pathology	Local tissue inflammation and dysfunction of upper airway because of type I, IgE-mediated hypersensitivity response.

case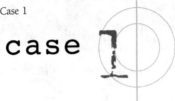

Allergic Rhinitis

Differential
Chronic Bronchitis
Emphysema
Foreign Body Aspiration
Mixed Connective-Tissue Disease
Sinusitis

Discussion
Allergic rhinitis is commonly caused by exposure to **pollens,** dust content, and insect matter; symptoms are mediated by the release of vasoactive and chemotactic mediators from mast cells and basophils (e.g., histamine and leukotrienes) with IgE surface receptors.

Treatment
Oral decongestants with intranasal corticosteroids; antihistamines; intranasal cromolyn sodium, especially before anticipated contact with allergen.

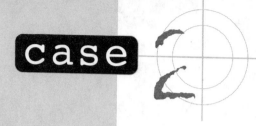

ID/CC   A 30-year-old woman presents to the ER with **severe, sudden-onset shortness of breath** and an **extensive** pruritic **skin rash.**

HPI   She was **prescribed cotrimoxazole** by her general physician for a UTI; she took the **first dose only a few minutes before** developing symptoms.

PE   VS: **hypotension.** PE: severe **respiratory distress;** central cyanosis; extensive **urticarial wheals** noted all over body.

Labs   **IgE antibody** demonstrated to sulfonamides by **RAST.**

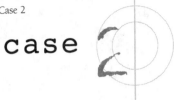

case 2

Anaphylaxis

Differential	Angioedema Malignant Carcinoid Syndrome Systemic Mastocytosis Pheochromocytoma Medullary Carcinoma of the Thyroid
Discussion	Systemic anaphylaxis is the most serious and life-threatening **IgE-mediated type I hypersensitivity reaction**; its recognition and prompt treatment are critical to survival.

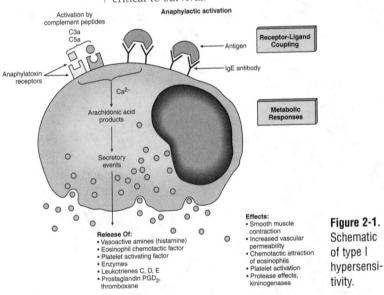

Figure 2-1. Schematic of type I hypersensitivity.

Release Of:
- Vasoactive amines (histamine)
- Eosinophil chemotactic factor
- Platelet activating factor
- Enzymes
- Leukotrienes C, D, E
- Prostaglandin PGD_2, thromboxane

Effects:
- Smooth muscle contraction
- Increased vascular permeability
- Chemotactic attraction of eosinophils
- Platelet activation
- Protease effects, kininogenases

Breakout Point

Hypersensitivity Reactions

Type I – Anaphylactic and Atopic (IgE mediated)
Type II – Cytotoxic or Cellular Dysfunction (IgG or IgM mediated)
Type III – Immune Complex Deposition (Antigen/Antibody Complexes)
Type IV – Delayed Type Hypersensitivity (T-lymphocyte mediated)

Treatment	Subcutaneous or IM **epinephrine** (1:1000); antihistaminics; steroids; ventilatory support; adequate IV fluid administration or vasopressor agents to treat hypotension.

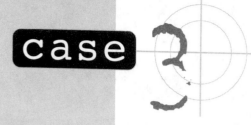

ID/CC A 3-year-old **albino** man is referred to a specialist for an evaluation of a suspected immune deficiency.

HPI His parents report **recurrent** respiratory, skin, and oral **infections with gram-negative and gram-positive** organisms. He also has a history of bruising easily.

PE **Partial albinism**; light-brown hair with silvery tint; **nystagmus; photophobia** on eye reflex exam; chronic gingivitis and periodontitis; purpuric patches over areas of repeated minimal trauma; mild hepatomegaly; no lymphadenopathy.

Labs CBC/PBS: **decreased neutrophil count** with normal platelet count; **large cytoplasmic granules** (GIANT LYSOSOMES) in WBCs on Wright-stained peripheral blood smears. Prolonged bleeding time; impaired platelet aggregation; normal clotting time and PTT; normal nitroblue tetrazolium test.

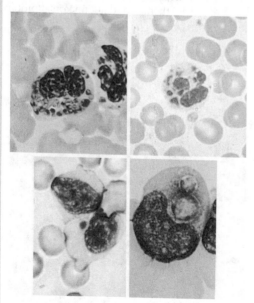

Figure 3-1. Multiple giant lysosomes in neutrophils.

case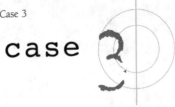

Chédiak-Higashi Syndrome

Differential

Albinism
Cutaneous T-Cell Lymphoma
Pyoderma Gangrenosum
Chronic Granulomatous Disease

Discussion

Chédiak-Higashi syndrome is an **autosomal-recessive** disorder that is due to a **defect in polymerization of microtubules in leukocytes** that causes impairment of chemotaxis, phagocytosis, and formation of phagolysosomes. Patients with this disorder usually present with **recurrent pyogenic staphylococcal and streptococcal infections.**

Treatment

Bone marrow transplantation is curative if attempted prior to development of accelerated phase; acyclovir, ascorbic acid, IV gamma globulin, vincristine, or interferon may be tried during accelerated phase; supportive therapy and antimicrobial prophylaxis.

case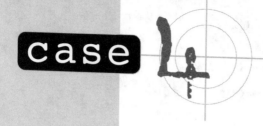

ID/CC A **2-year-old boy** is admitted to the hospital for evaluation of a suspected immune disorder.

HPI He has a history of **recurrent fungal** diaper rashes and **staphylococcal cervical furunculosis** requiring multiple incisions and drainage in addition to antibiotics. His mother also reports chronic diarrhea and a prior perianal fistula.

PE Cervical lymphadenopathy; mild hepatomegaly and splenomegaly; no pallor, purpuric patches, or sternal tenderness.

Labs CBC/PBS: **neutrophilic leukocytosis.** Elevated ESR; normal serum immunoglobulins; nitroblue tetrazolium test demonstrates low phagocytic oxidase activity.

Imaging CXR: hilar lymphadenopathy. US, abdomen: hepatosplenomegaly; hepatic and splenic nodular lesions (due to granulomas).

Micro Pathology Characteristic granuloma formation with phagocytes, giant cells, and occasional histiocytes in lymph nodes, liver, spleen, and lungs.

case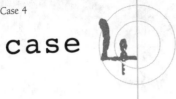

Chronic Granulomatous Disease

Differential	Bruton Agammaglobulinemia
	Common Variable Immunodeficiency
	HIV Infection
	Hyperimmunoglobulinemia E (Job) Syndrome
	Leukocyte Adhesion Deficiency
Discussion	Chronic granulomatous disease is most commonly an **X-linked** disorder of neutrophil function (may have variable inheritance patterns) that is due to a **deficiency of NADPH oxidase**. Neutrophils of affected patients demonstrate normal chemotaxis, degranulation, and phagocytosis but cannot use the oxygen-dependent myeloperoxidase system for microbial killing, making patients susceptible to recurrent staphylococcal infections.

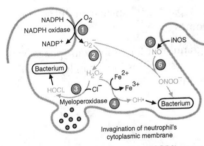

Figure 4-1. Production of reactive oxygen species during the phagocytic respiratory burst by activated neutrophils. (1) Activation of NADPH oxidase on the outer side of the plasma membrane initiates the respiratory burst with the generation of superoxide. During the phagocytosis, the plasma membrane invaginates, so superoxide is released into the vacuole space. (2) Superoxide (either spontaneously or enzymatically via superoxide dismutase [SOD]) generates hydrogen peroxide (H_2O_2). (3) Granules containing myeloperoxidase are secreted into the phagosome, where myeloperoxidase generates hypochlorous acid (HOCl) and other halides. (4) H_2O_2 can also generate the hydroxyl radical from the Fenton reaction. (5) Inducible nitric oxide synthase may be activated and generate NO. (6) Nitric oxide combines with superoxide to form peroxynitrite, which may generate additional reactive nitrogen oxide species (RNOS). The result is an attack on the membranes and other components of phagocytosed cells, and eventual lysis. The whole process is referred to as the respiratory burst because it lasts only 30 to 60 minutes and consumes oxygen (O_2).

Breakout Point

Superoxide is the most potent antimicrobial defense a neutrophil possesses. There are patients who have defects in the myeloperoxidase enzyme; however, this is usually unappreciated clinically.

Treatment	Long-term TMP-SMX prophylaxis, γ-interferon.

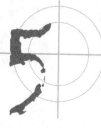

case 5

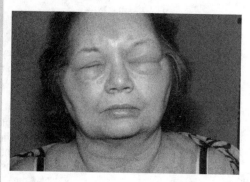

ID/CC A 49-year-old woman has **recurrent attacks** of bilateral **periorbital and hand swelling** coupled with **respiratory difficulty that lasts up to 24 hours** and often requires hospitalization.

Figure 5-1. Bilateral periorbital edema.

HPI She does not, however, complain of itching. Her **father** and her **aunt** both suffer from a **similar illness**.

PE Physical examination unremarkable.

Labs **Decreased C4** (best screening test); **decreased C1 inhibitor** (confirmatory test) and C2; normal C3; normal IgE.

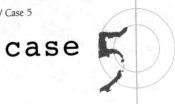

case 5

Hereditary Angioedema

Differential

Anaphylaxis
Asthma
Epiglottitis
Peritonsillar Abscess
Ludwig Angina

Discussion

C1 esterase inhibitor deficiency is inherited as an **autosomal-dominant** trait; **death** may result from **laryngeal edema.** Also known as hereditary angioedema.

Breakout Point

> Another defect in the complement system is a defect in the formation of the C5–9 (membrane attack) complex. Such patients are susceptible to recurrent *Neisseria* infections.

Treatment

Vapor-heated C1 esterase inhibitor concentrate for acute attacks; synthetic androgens (e.g., danazol) or aminocaproic acid for prophylaxis.

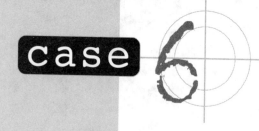

ID/CC A 25-year-old **White** woman is referred to an internist by her family doctor for a workup of **recurrent sinusitis**, chronic otitis media, one episode of **pneumonia** that required hospitalization, and recurrent bouts of watery **diarrhea**.

HPI She has seen an allergy specialist for several years and has received desensitization shots for **multiple allergies**, including pollen, dust, and cat hair.

PE Normal except for **hypopigmented spots on neck and arms** (VITILIGO).

Labs **Markedly decreased serum IgA; normal IgG and IgM.**

Imaging XR, sinus: opacification of paranasal sinuses (due to chronic sinusitis).

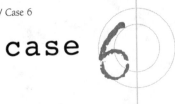

case 6

Selective Immunoglobulin A Deficiency

Differential

Combined B-Cell and T-Cell Disorders
Severe Combined Immunodeficiency
Wiskott-Aldrich Syndrome

Discussion

Selective IgA deficiency is the **most common congenital immunodeficiency**, especially in patients of European descent. Diarrhea is usually caused by *Giardia lamblia*; recurrent sinopulmonary infections are caused by *Streptococcus pneumoniae, Haemophilus influenzae*, or *Staphylococcus aureus*; associated with an increased incidence of allergies and autoimmune diseases such as SLE and rheumatoid arthritis. Selective IgA deficiency may be due to a specific defect in isotype switching.

▪ TABLE 6-1 PRIMARY HUMORAL IMMUNODEFICIENCY DISORDERS

Disease	Mode of Inheritance[a]	Locus/Gene
Agammaglobulinemia	XL	Xq21.3/*BTK*
Selective antibody class/ subclass deficiencies		
γ1 isotype	AR	14q32.33
γ2 isotype	AR	14q32.33
Partial γ3 isotype	AR	14q32.33
γ4 isotype	AR	14q32.33
IgG subclass ± IgA deficiency	?	—
α1 isotype	AR	14q32.33
α2 isotype	AR	14q32.33
ε isotype	AR	14q32.33
IgA deficiency	Varied	—
Common variable immunodeficiency	Varied	—

[a]XL, X-linked; AR, autosomal recessive.

Breakout Point

> Patients with selective IgA are susceptible to anaphylaxis with blood or plasma transfusions.

Treatment

Largely supportive; antibiotic therapy; pneumococcal vaccination; try to **avoid blood or plasma transfusion** (anaphylaxis or serum sickness due to presence of antibodies to IgA).

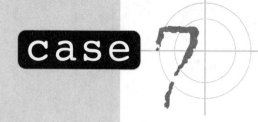

ID/CC A **4-month-old baby boy** presents with **chronic diarrhea** and **failure to thrive**.

HPI The infant was diagnosed with extensive **mucocutaneous candidiasis** in the early neonatal period and shortly thereafter developed a fulminant *Pseudomonas* **septicemia** that required intravenous antibiotic therapy for an extended period of time. A paternal cousin had developed similar and equally devastating bacterial and fungal infections in the neonatal period and subsequently died.

PE Emaciated; mucocutaneous **candidiasis** noted; **tonsils not seen; lymph nodes not palpable** despite recurrent infections.

Labs CBC: severe lymphopenia. PBS: **lack of mature lymphocytes.** Tests for cutaneous **delayed hypersensitivity** and contact sensitization negative; **serum immunoglobulin levels** (IgG, IgA, and IgM) **low.**

Imaging CXR: **absent thymic shadow.**

Gross Pathology Thymus fails to descend into the anterior mediastinum from the neck and resembles fetal thymus of 6 to 8 weeks.

Micro Pathology No lymphoid tissue in the lymph nodes, spleen, tonsils, and appendix.

case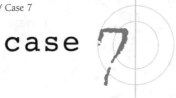

Severe Combined Immunodeficiency

Differential | Wiskott-Aldrich Syndrome
HIV Infection
Hyperimmunoglobulinemia E (Job) Syndrome
Lymphohistiocytosis
Lymphoproliferative Disorders

Discussion | SCID is characterized by marked depletion of the cells that mediate both humoral (B-cell) and cellular (T-cell) immunity. SCID may be transmitted as either an autosomal-recessive trait or an X-linked recessive trait, or it may be sporadic; half of the cases inherited in an **autosomal-recessive** manner are caused by a **deficiency in ADA.**

■ TABLE 7-1 TEN ABNORMAL GENES IN SCID

Cytokine Receptor Genes
IL2RG
JAK3
IL7Rα
Antigen Receptor Genes
RAG1
RAG2
ARTEMIS
CD3δ and ε
Other Genes
ADA
CD45

Treatment | **Bone marrow transplant** from an HLA-identical sibling; IV Ig; antibiotics; gene therapy for ADA; genetic counseling (SCID caused by ADA deficiency can be diagnosed prenatally by amniocentesis).

Breakout Point |

> ADA SCID was the first disorder for which human gene therapy has been successful.

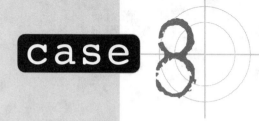

ID/CC   A 28-year-old man presents with a **red, pruritic skin eruption** on his trunk and his upper and lower limbs of a few hours' duration.

HPI   One day earlier, he was prescribed cotrimoxazole for a UTI. He has not experienced any dyspnea.

PE   Erythematous, warm, wheals (hives) seen over trunk, legs, and arms; no angioedema or respiratory distress.

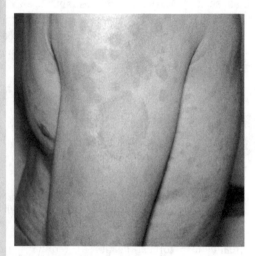

Figure 8-1. Wheals over the trunk and arms.

Labs   CBC: leukocytosis with eosinophilia. No parasites revealed on stool exam.

Gross Pathology   Linear or oval, **raised papules or plaque-like wheals** up to several centimeters in diameter.

Micro Pathology   Wide separation of dermal collagen fibers with dilatation of lymphatics and venules.

case 8

Urticaria

Differential

Bullous Pemphigoid

Dermatitis Herpetiformis

Chronic Pruritus (nonurticarial)

Hypersensitivity Vasculitis

Pruritic Urticarial Papules and Plaques of Pregnancy (PUPPP)

Discussion

Mast cells and basophils are focal to urticarial reaction. When stimulated by certain immunologic or nonimmunologic mechanisms, storage granules in these cells release histamine and other mediators, such as kinins and leukotrienes. These agents produce the localized vasodilatation and transudation of fluid that characterize urticaria.

Breakout Point

Urticaria Display a Typical "Triple Response of Lewis"

1. Erythema – vasodilation
2. Wheal – vascular leakage
3. Pruritis – release of bradykinin

Treatment

Topical agents to reduce itching; avoidance of causative agent (in this case, cotrimoxazole); antihistamines (primarily H_1 blockers but also H_2 blockers); consider glucocorticoids.

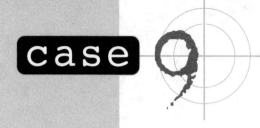

ID/CC   A 2-year-old **boy** is brought to his pediatrician because of recurrent **epistaxis** and chronic **eczematous dermatitis**.

HPI   He has a history of **recurring pneumonia** and bilateral **chronic** suppurative **otitis media**. A **male cousin** suffers from a **similar illness**.

PE   Epistaxis; eczematous dermatitis over both legs; several **purpuric patches** over skin; mild splenomegaly and cervical lymphadenopathy.

Labs   CBC/PBS: **thrombocytopenia;** lymphopenia. Decreased isohemagglutinins; decreased IgM; increased IgE, normal IgG, and increased IgA; **inability to form IgM antibody to carbohydrate antigens** (i.e., capsular polysaccharides of bacteria).

case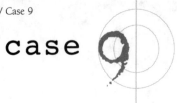

Wiskott-Aldrich Syndrome

Differential

Agammaglobulinemia

Atopic Dermatitis

Bruton Agammaglobulinemia

DiGeorge Syndrome

Severe Combined Immunodeficiency

Discussion

Wiskott–Aldrich syndrome is a rare **X-linked recessive** disease with **B-cell deficiency and T-cell deficiency** characterized by a **triad of thrombocytopenia, eczema, and recurrent pyogenic infections**; it is due to a deletion of the Wiskott-Aldrich syndrome protein (WASP) gene in the p11 region of the X chromosome. The condition is associated with an increased incidence of **lymphomas**.

Breakout Point

> Wiskott-Aldrich Syndrome:
> thrombocytopenia, eczema, and recurrent infection

Treatment

Largely supportive; IVIG; bone marrow transplant; splenectomy.

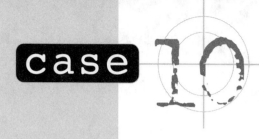

ID/CC A 7-month-old **baby boy** is admitted for a workup of **recurrent upper respiratory tract and skin infections** of several months' duration.

HPI His parents state that he has had recurrent URIs, one episode of *Haemophilus influenzae* **pneumonia**, and severe otitis media.

PE Low weight and height for chronological age; chronic bilateral suppurative otitis media; **asymmetric arthritis** of knees; **no tonsillar tissue** seen; no lymphadenopathy or hepatosplenomegaly.

Labs **Panhypogammaglobulinemia: very low** IgG; IgA and IgM undetectable.

case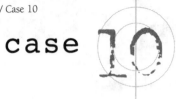

X-Linked Hypogammaglobulinemia

Differential

Aplastic Anemia

Hypogammaglobulinemia

Infectious Mononucleosis

Lymphoma

Cystic Fibrosis

Discussion

An X-linked disease (manifests **only in males**) characterized by a **selective B-cell defect** with **recurrent bacterial infections.** Also known as **Bruton disease,** X-linked hypogammaglobulinemia is due to a genetic defect in tyrosine kinase receptor found on antibody precursors, resulting in impaired maturation and development of antibodies. Male infants demonstrate infections when maternal antibodies have cleared from their system.

Breakout Point

X-linked Immunodeficiency Syndromes:
SCID Wiskott-Aldrich Syndrome Bruton Agammaglobulinemia Chronic Granulomatatous Disease

Treatment

IVIG; antibiotics; monitor pulmonary function to guard against chronic lung disease.

case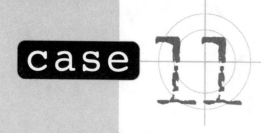

ID/CC A 48-year-old missionary who has lived in Cameroon, **West Africa,** for 20 years is airlifted home because of lethargy, nuchal rigidity, persistent headache, and drowsiness that have not responded to antibiotics and supportive treatment.

HPI He states that over the years he has been bitten in the neck several times by a mutumutu, or **tsetse fly** (*Glossina palpalis*). He has also had intermittent, generalized erythematous rashes accompanied by fever.

PE Alert but somewhat **incoherent and confused;** sometimes delusional; nuchal rigidity and **tremors of face and lips;** splenomegaly; generalized **rubbery, painless lymphadenopathy,** predominantly in posterior neck and supraclavicular areas (WINTERBOTTOM SIGN).

Labs PBS/LP: hypercellular, **trypanosomal** forms present; lymphocytes in CSF. **Elevated IgM.**

Gross Pathology Chancre with erythema and induration at bite site; chancre resolves spontaneously; spleen and lymph nodes enlarged during systemic stage; leptomeninges enlarged during CNS involvement.

Micro Pathology Skin: edema, mononuclear cell inflammation, organisms, and endothelial proliferation; spleen and lymph nodes: histiocytic hyperplasia; CNS: mononuclear cell meningoencephalitis.

case 11

African Trypanosomiasis

Differential

Malaria
HIV Infection
Brucellosis
Tuberculosis
Babesia microti Infection

Discussion

Also called **sleeping sickness,** African trypanosomiasis is a systemic febrile disease endemic to Africa whose chronic form causes a meningoencephalitis. It is caused by the flagellated protozoans *Trypanosoma brucei gambiense* (West African) and *Trypanosoma brucei rhodesiense* (East African), which are transmitted by the tsetse fly.

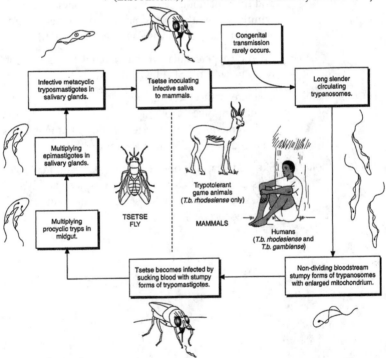

Figure 11-1. Differentiation in mammals of the longitudinally dividing slender bloodstream trypanosomes, preadapted for infecting tsetse flies.

Treatment

Suramin; pentamidine or eflornithine.

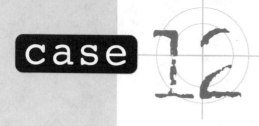

case 12

ID/CC	A 28-year-old man from **India** complains of gradual-onset, intermittent, **crampy abdominal pain** with 1 to 4 **foul-smelling, frothy loose stools daily.**
HPI	His stools sometimes contain blood and mucus. He also complains of flatulence, tenesmus, and, at times, alternating diarrhea and constipation.
PE	Slight tenderness during palpation of cecum and ascending colon; no hepatomegaly.
Labs	CBC: mild leukocytosis; no eosinophilia. Fresh stool examination reveals presence **of cysts and motile hematophagous trophozoites.**
Imaging	Colonoscopy: **multiple colonic mucosal ulcers** that are slightly raised and covered with shaggy exudate; mucosa between ulcers normal.
Micro Pathology	Biopsy specimens reveal lesions extending under adjacent intact mucosa to produce classical **"flask-shaped" ulcers;** amebic trophozoites demonstrated at base of ulcer.

PARASITOLOGY

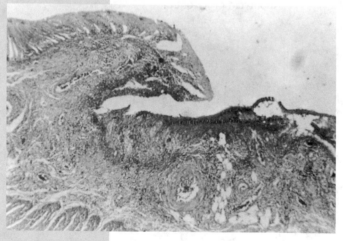

Figure 12-1. Flask-shaped ulcer.

case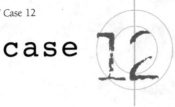

Amebic Colitis

Differential
Abdominal Abscess
Arteriovenous Malformation
Diverticulosis
Enterotoxigenic *Escherichia coli*
Shigellosis

Discussion
Entamoeba histolytica cysts are infective and are transmitted through contaminated water, raw vegetables, food handlers, and fecal-oral or oral-anal contact. The sites of involvement, in order of frequency, are the cecum and ascending colon, rectum, sigmoid colon, appendix, and terminal ileum. Trophozoites are the invasive form of the organism, causing colitis or distant infection by hematogenous spread. Complications include perforation of the bowel; liver abscess with pleural, pericardial, or peritoneal rupture; bowel obstruction by ameboma; and skin ulcers around the perineum and genitalia.

Treatment
Metronidazole (drug of choice) followed by paromomycin or iodoquinol.

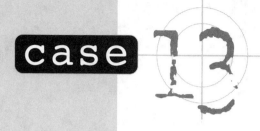

ID/CC A 45-year-old man Peace Corps volunteer who recently spent 2 years in rural Mexico complains of a **spiking fever,** malaise, headache, and **RUQ abdominal pain.**

HPI He admits to having had **bloody diarrhea with mucus** (DYSENTERY) and tenesmus that disappeared with some pills that he took several months ago.

PE VS: fever (39.6°C). PE: pallor; slight jaundice; tender **hepatomegaly** with no rebound tenderness; pain on fist percussion of right lower ribs.

Labs CBC: leukocytosis with neutrophilia. Amebic cysts in stool specimen (not concurrent with abscess).

Imaging CXR: elevation of right hemidiaphragm; small right pleural effusion. CT/US: cavitating lesion in **right lobe of liver** (due to abscess).

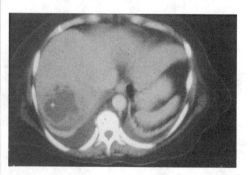

Figure 13-1. Computed tomography with oral contrast shows a hypodense lesion in the right lobe of the liver.

Gross Pathology Multiple colonic mucosal ulcers, slightly raised and covered with shaggy exudate; enlarged liver with **one large abscess** on right lobe containing chocolate-colored pus; abscess may rupture and spread to lungs, brain, or other organs.

Micro Pathology Sterile pus; ameba may be obtained from periphery of lesion.

PARASITOLOGY

25

case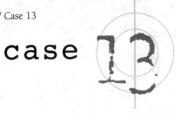

Amebic Liver Abscess

Differential
Biliary Disease
Echinococcosis Hydatid Cyst
Hepatocellular carcinoma
Hydatid Cyst
Malaria
Typhoid fever

Discussion
Prior travel to endemic areas plus a triad of fever, hepatomegaly, and RUQ pain are hallmarks of hepatic liver abscess. Colitis precedes the liver abscess; amebas then invade the gut wall and enter portal circulation.

Treatment
Metronidazole; needle evacuation; surgery in case of treatment failure or rupture.

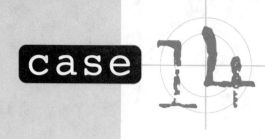

case 14

ID/CC	A **15-year-old boy** who resides in Florida presents with **nausea** and vomiting, **fever**, and **marked neck stiffness**.
HPI	He also complains of a severe bifrontal headache. Careful history reveals that he **swam for several hours in brackish water** approximately a week ago.
PE	VS: fever; tachycardia. PE: signs of meningeal irritation (neck rigidity, positive Kernig sign and Brudzinski sign); funduscopy reveals mild papilledema.
Labs	LP: bloody CSF (raised RBC count may also be due to examiner's inability to recognize proliferating amebas) shows intense neutrophilia, pleocytosis, high protein, and low sugar; no organism seen on Gram, ZN, or India-ink staining of CSF; **wet preparation** of CSF reveals viable amebas; diagnosis confirmed using direct fluorescent antibody staining.
Gross Pathology	Lesions are mostly present in the olfactory nerves and brain. Focal hemorrhages, extensive fibrinoid necrosis, and blood vessel thrombosis with nerve tissue necrosis.
Micro Pathology	Trophozoites seen as 10-μm-diameter to 20-μm-diameter organisms with large nucleus, small granular cytoplasm, distinct ectoplasm, and bulbous pseudopodia.

case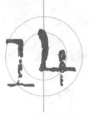

Amebic Meningoencephalitis

Differential
Echinococcosis
Malaria
Aseptic Meningitis
Bacterial Meningitis
Rabies
Toxoplasmosis
Tuberculosis

Discussion
Primary amebic meningoencephalitis is caused by amebas of the genus *Naegleria* or *Acanthamoeba*. The former most often affects children and young adults; appears to be acquired by swimming in warm, fresh/brackish water; and is almost always fatal, with the ameba gaining entry into the arachnoid space through the nasal cribriform plate. *Acanthamoeba* infections involve older, immunocompromised individuals and are sometimes characterized by spontaneous recovery.

Treatment
Intracisternal and IV **amphotericin B** with adjunctive rifampin and doxycycline; prognosis is poor.

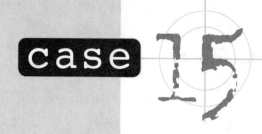
ID/CC A 35-year-old **Finnish** man complains of **easy fatigability and shortness of breath.**

HPI He often eats **undercooked or raw freshwater fish.** He also reports vague digestive disturbances such as anorexia, heartburn, and nausea.

PE PE: pallor.

Labs CBC/PBS: **megaloblastic anemia.** Blood **vitamin B_{12} levels low;** stool exam reveals presence of **operculated eggs and proglottids.**

PARASITOLOGY

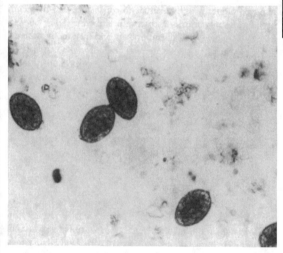

Figure 15-1. Operculated ovoids in stool sample.

case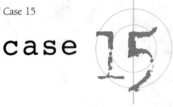

Anemia—*Diphyllobothrium Latum*

Differential

Pernicious Anemia
Dietary Deficiency
Taenia Infection
Chronic Anemia
Short-Gut Syndrome
Anticonvulsant Use

Discussion

Diphyllobothrium latum (fish tapeworm) infection is found in cold climates where **raw or undercooked fish** are eaten. The adult worm attaches to the human jejunum and **competes for absorption of vitamin B_{12},** producing a deficiency that resembles pernicious anemia. Prevention includes proper preparation of fish.

Treatment

Niclosamide or praziquantel.

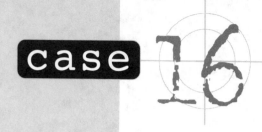

ID/CC   An 8-year-old White girl enters the ER complaining of headache, malaise, and bipalpebral **swelling of the right eye.**

HPI   She recently returned from a year-long stay in **Brazil,** where her father works as a logger in the **Amazon forest.** Over the past week she had a high fever, which was treated at home as malaria.

PE   VS: fever (39°C); tachycardia. PE: right eyelid swollen shut (ROMAÑA SIGN); markedly hyperemic conjunctiva; **ipsilateral retroauricular and cervical lymph nodes;** hepatosplenomegaly.

Labs   PBS: **trypanosomes on thick blood smear.** ECG: right bundle-branch block; ventricular extrasystoles.

PARASITOLOGY

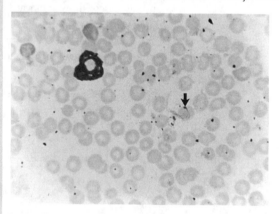

Figure 16-1. C-shaped configuration of parasite found in human blood.

Gross Pathology   Encapsulated, nodular area or Romaña sign may be seen at point of entry, commonly the face.

Micro Pathology   Intense neutrophilic infiltrate with abundant macrophages at site of entry; myocardial necrosis with mononuclear cell infiltration; pseudocysts in infected tissues contain parasites that multiply within cells; denervation of myenteric gut plexus.

31

case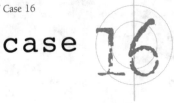

Chagas Disease

Differential

Hypertrophic Cardiomyopathy

Esophageal Cancer

Leishmaniasis

Malaria

Toxoplasmosis

GERD

Discussion

Chagas disease is a parasitic disease that is restricted to the Americas (endemic in South and Central America) and is produced by *Trypanosoma cruzi*, a thin, undulating flagellated protozoan; it is transmitted by contamination of a **reduviid bug** bite by injection of its feces. Also known as American trypanosomiasis. Longstanding cases show myocardial involvement with **dilated cardiomyopathy,** life-threatening conduction defects, and apical aneurysm formation and may also show **megaesophagus or megacolon.**

Breakout Point

> Chagas disease is the most frequent cause of heart failure in Latin America.

Treatment

Nifurtimox for acute disease.

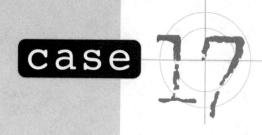

case 17

ID/CC	A 30-year-old man with **AIDS** presents with chronic, recurrent **profuse, nonbloody, watery diarrhea.**
HPI	The diarrhea has recurred over the past 2 months with intermittent cramping, and previous treatments have not been effective.
PE	VS: no fever. PS: moderate **dehydration;** thin; generalized lymphadenopathy.
Labs	**Acid-fast** staining demonstrates oocysts in fresh stool.

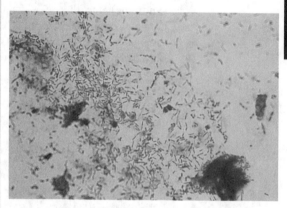

Figure 17-1. Ziehl-Nielsen (ZN) stain of stool specimen showing acid-fast oocysts.

Gross Pathology	Intestinal mucosa appears normal.
Micro Pathology	Blunting of intestinal villi; mixed inflammatory cell infiltrates with eosinophils in lamina propria; organisms visible on brush borders.

33

case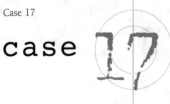

Cryptosporidiosis

Differential

Amebiasis
Campylobacter Infection
CMV Infection
Giardiasis
Isosporiasis
Salmonellosis

Discussion

Cryptosporidium parvum infection presents as acute diarrhea in malnourished children and as severe diarrhea in immunocompromised patients (part of **HIV wasting syndrome**); the disease is mild and self-limiting in immune-competent patients. The disease is acquired through the ingestion of oocysts (fecal-oral transmission) that may be **killed by chlorination.**

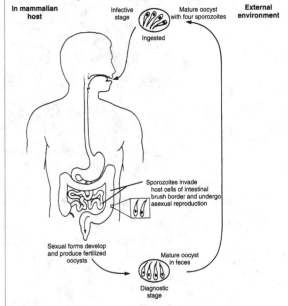

Figure 17-2. Life cycle of *Cryptosporidium* species.

Treatment

No treatment found effective; paromomycin may limit diarrhea; supportive management with maintenance of fluids and nutrition.

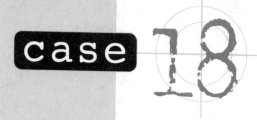

case 18

ID/CC A 43-year-old man, a **Mexican** migrant worker visits his ophthalmologist because of pain and **loss of vision** in his right eye.

HPI Recently he has also suffered from **severe headaches** and **projectile vomiting**.

PE **Papilledema** on left funduscopic exam; **free-floating cyst** in vitreous body of right eye; chorioretinitis and disk hemorrhage; multiple nontender subcutaneous nodules.

Labs CBC: eosinophilia. LP: lymphocytic and eosinophilic pleocytosis in CSF with elevated protein and decreased glucose. Eggs of *Taenia solium* in stool sample.

Imaging XR, plain: small nodular calcifications. CT/MR imaging, brain: characteristic ring-enhancing **intracranial** cysts or calcifications, can cause obstruction and hydrocephalus.

Gross Pathology Fluid-filled cysts containing scolex surrounded by fibrous capsule in anterior chamber of eye; intraventricular and parenchymal invasion of brain, subcutaneous tissue, and striated muscle.

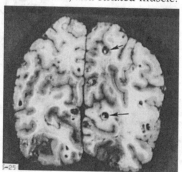

Figure 18-1. Coronal section of human brain showing multiple parenchymatous calcified cysts *(arrows)*.

Micro Pathology Inflammatory infiltration of cyst by PMN leukocytes; necrotic inflammation with calcification upon death of parasite.

35

case 18

Cysticercosis

Differential | Brain Abscess
Tuberculoma
CNS Neoplasm
Meningitis
Encephalitis

Discussion | Produced by *Cysticercus cellulosae*, the larval form of the pork tapeworm *Taenia solium*, neurocysticercosis is due to the ingestion of ova and spreads through fecal-oral transmission.

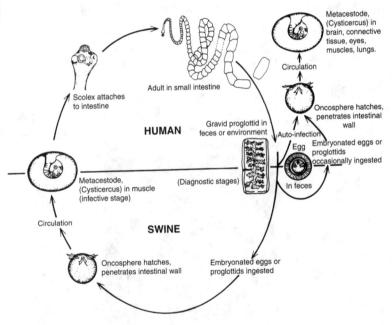

Figure 18-2. Life cycle of *Taenia solium*.

Treatment | Surgical removal of parasite from eye; albendazole, corticosteroids/praziquantel for brain disease.

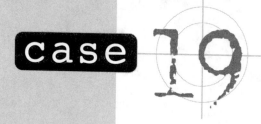

ID/CC	A 56-year-old man, a professor of veterinary medicine from **New Zealand** experiences sudden **high fever** with chills, **jaundice**, and **RUQ pain** while attending a conference in the United States.
HPI	His past history is unremarkable. He has been healthy and has been physically active working in the field with sheep and breeding **dogs**.
PE	VS: fever; hypotension (BP 90/50). PE: **hepatomegaly;** jaundiced sclera; on palpation of epigastrium and right hypochondrium, abdomen is tender with no rebound tenderness.
Labs	CBC: leukocytosis with neutrophilia; slight eosinophilia. Elevated direct bilirubin and alkaline phosphatase.
Imaging	CT/US, abdomen: **multiple large septated liver cysts** impinging on bile ducts, producing biliary dilatation (due to obstruction).

PARASITOLOGY

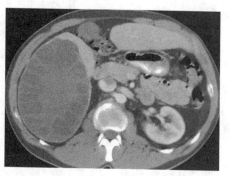

Figure 19-1. Contrast-enhanced CT image shows a large multilocular mass with a thick wall. Multiple daughter cysts line the periphery of the mass.

Gross Pathology	Liver is most common site of invasion, but cysts may also form in lungs, kidneys, bones, and brain; each cyst contains millions of scoleces.
Micro Pathology	Giant cell reaction surrounding cyst with eosinophilic infiltration.

case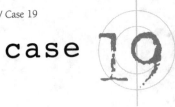

Echinococcosis

Differential | Amebic Hepatic Abscess
Biliary Disease
Budd-Chiari Syndrome
Cysticercosis
Schistosomiasis

Discussion | Echinococcosis is a zoonosis produced by *Echinococcus granulosus*. It is acquired through the ingestion of food or drink contaminated with the **feces of dogs** or other carnivores that have **eaten contaminated meat**; humans are the intermediate host of parasitic larvae. Accidental spilling of cyst fluid, either spontaneously or during surgery, may result in secondary seeding or anaphylaxis and even death. Also known as **hydatid disease**.

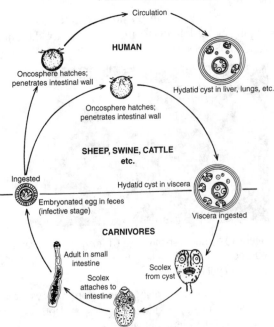

Figure 19-2. Life cycle of *Echinococcus granulosus*.

Treatment | Surgically remove cysts if possible; albendazole may be effective.

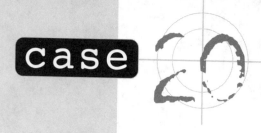
ID/CC A 4-year-old girl is brought to the pediatrician because of **lack of appetite**; nausea and **vomiting**; **chronic, foul-smelling diarrhea** without blood or mucus; and a **bloated** sensation.

HPI She has been in several **day-care centers** over the past 3 years.

PE **Low weight and height** for age; mild epigastric tenderness.

Labs **Binucleate, pear-shaped, flagellated trophozoites** on freshly passed stool; cysts found on stool exam.

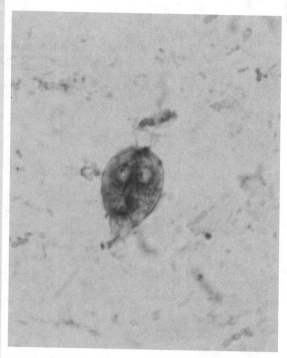

Figure 20-1. Binucleate, pear-shaped, flagellated trophozoite.

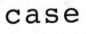 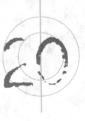

Giardiasis

Differential
: Amebiasis
Crohn Disease
Cryptosporidium Infection
Celiac Sprue
Irritable Bowel Syndrome

Discussion
: Giardiasis is transmitted mainly through **contaminated food or water** and causes malabsorption. If stool ova and parasite examination is negative, **string test** may show trophozoites from duodenum or, alternatively, a stool antigen detection test for *Giardia* may be used.

Breakout Point

> *Giardia lamblia* is **the most** common protozoal infection in children in the United States.

Treatment
: Metronidazole.

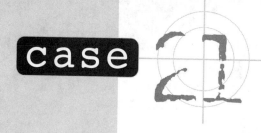

ID/CC A 10-year-old man complains of generalized weakness, faintness on exertion, and occasional epigastric pain.

HPI His mother has noticed that he often **eats soil and other inedible things** (PICA).

PE Pallor; puffy face and dependent edema.

Labs CBC: **microcytic, hypochromic anemia; eosinophilia. Low serum iron and ferritin;** elevated serum transferrin; reduced bone marrow hemosiderin; **hypoproteinemia;** stool exam revealed ovoid eggs with thin transparent shell that reveal the segmented embryo within.

Micro Pathology Section of the ileum shows two portions of an adult worm with a **mucosal plug in the buccal cavity of the worm.**

PARASITOLOGY

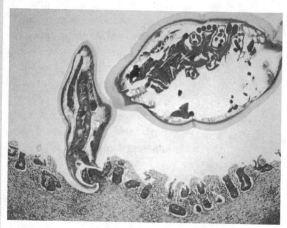

Figure 21-1. Pathology section of ileum.

case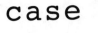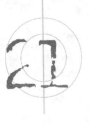

Hookworm Infection

Differential

Eosinophilia

Bacterial Gastroenteritis

Iron Deficiency Anemia

Plummer-Vinson Syndrome

Discussion

Infection with hookworms, either *Ancylostoma duodenale* or *Necator americanus*, is more likely where unsanitary conditions exist; individuals at risk include children, gardeners, plumbers, electricians, and armed-forces personnel who are in contact with soil. Hookworm eggs excreted in the feces hatch in the soil, releasing larvae that develop into infective larvae. Percutaneous larval penetration is the principal mode of human infection. From the skin, hookworm larvae travel via the bloodstream to the lungs, enter the alveoli, ascend the bronchotracheal tree to the pharynx, and are swallowed. Although transpulmonary larval passage may elicit a transient **eosinophilic pneumonitis** (LÖFFLER PNEUMONITIS), this phenomenon is much less common with hookworm infections than with roundworm infections. The major health impact of hookworm infection, however, is iron loss resulting from the 0.1 to 0.4 mL of blood ingested daily by each adult worm. In malnourished hosts, such blood loss can lead to **severe iron deficiency anemia.**

Breakout Point

> **Hookworm infections are the most common cause of chronic anemia worldwide.**

Treatment

Albendazole or mebendazole; **iron supplementation** to treat iron deficiency anemia.

case

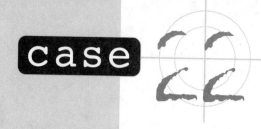

ID/CC A 57-year-old Black woman from Kenya complains of increasing weight and **edema of the lower legs** with difficulty walking.

HPI Over the years she has had episodes of **fever with swelling of inguinal lymph nodes** and itching. She has also had numerous attacks of malaria.

PE Inguinal lymph nodes indurated and slightly increased in size; marked deformity in both legs with **thickening of skin** and greatly **increased diameter; rubbery consistency.**

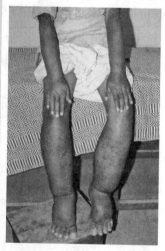

Figure 22-1. Bilateral swelling of the lower extremities.

Labs PBS: several **microfilariae**; prominent **eosinophilia.**

Imaging Lymphangiogram: partial lymphatic obstruction at iliac level.

Gross Pathology Presence of adult worms in lymphatics; marked fibrosis surrounding obstructed vessels.

Micro Pathology Granulomatous reaction with plasma cell and lymphocytic infiltration; giant cell formation; intense fibroblastic hyperplasia.

PARASITOLOGY

43

case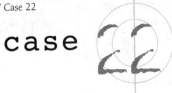

Lymphatic Filariasis

Differential

Lymphedema
Sporotrichosis
Lymphosarcoma
Leprosy
Lymphoma

Discussion

Lymphatic filariasis is a chronic disease that is due to lymphatic obstruction and is caused by several types of filarial roundworms, mainly *Wuchereria bancrofti* and *Brugia malayi*; it is transmitted by female **mosquito bites.** Also known as elephantiasis.

Treatment

Ivermectin; diethylcarbamazine; surgery in advanced cases.

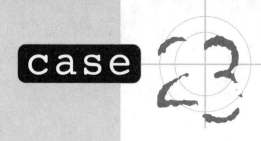

ID/CC A 30-year-old missionary comes to the ER complaining of **high fever, chills, severe headache,** and confusion.

HPI Upon returning from **Africa** 2 weeks ago, he began to feel weak and experienced backaches, pain behind the eyes, and sleepiness.

PE VS: fever (39°C); tachycardia. PE: pallor; profuse **sweating;** mild splenomegaly without lymphadenopathy.

Labs CBC/PBS: anemia; thrombocytopenia; **ring shaped gametocytes in erythrocytes on thick peripheral blood smear.** Slight hyperbilirubinemia and hypoglycemia.

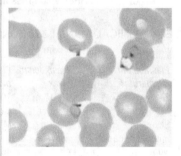

Figure 23-1. Ringed gametocytes within RBCs.

Gross Pathology Liver and spleen moderately enlarged and soft in con sistency, with sequestration and hemolysis of erythrocytes and macrophages; hyperplasia of Kupffer cells; malarial pigment in spleen and liver; brain capillaries may show thromboses.

Micro Pathology Hypertrophy of phagocytic system; ischemic necrosis surrounding occluded blood vessels in brain.

PARASITOLOGY

case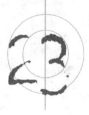

Malaria

Differential

African Trypanosomiasis
Dengue Fever
Leptospirosis
Infectious Mononucleosis

Discussion

Malaria is transmitted by female *Anopheles* **mosquitoes**. *Plasmodium falciparum* may be lethal, producing cerebral malaria. Other types include *Plasmodium vivax*, *Plasmodium ovale*, and *Plasmodium malariae*.

Breakout Point

> **Blackwater fever,** a manifestation of *Plasmodium falciparum* infection, is due to massive hemolysis of infected RBCs with **gross hemoglobinuria.**

■ TABLE 23-1 SELECT CLINICAL MANIFESTATIONS OF FOUR TYPES OF MALARIA

Characteristic	Plasmodium falciparum	Plasmodium vivax	Plasmodium ovale	Plasmodium malariae
Usual incubation period (d)	8–11	10–17 or longer	10–17 or longer	18–40 or longer
Severity of primary attack	Severe in nonimmune	Mild to severe	Mild	Mild
Periodicity (h)	None	48	48	72
Duration of untreated primary attack (wk)	2–3	3–8	2–3	3–24
Duration of untreated infection	6–17 mo	5–7 yr	12 mo	20+ yr
Average parasitemia (per mm^2)	≥20,000	10,000	9,000	6,000
Anemia	Frequent and severe	Mild	Mild	Mild
CNS involvement	Yes, severe	Rare	Rare	Rare
Nephritic syndrome	Rare	Rare	No	Frequent

d, days; h, hours; wk, weeks; mo, months; yr, years; CNS, central nervous system.

Treatment

Chloroquine; doxycycline, pyrimethamine/sulfadoxine, mefloquine, quinine, or atovaquone/proguanil for chloroquine-resistant infection; primaquine for radical treatment.

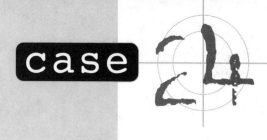

case

ID/CC A 56-year-old White woman is referred to an ophthalmologist for an evaluation of **diminished visual acuity.**

HPI She has spent most of her adult life as a missionary in rural **Senegal** and **Mali.** She admits to chronic **generalized itching, mostly while showering.**

PE Wrinkling and loss of elastic tissue in skin; **marked hypopigmentation of shins;** 2-cm to 3-cm, nonfixed, firm, nontender subcutaneous **nodules on iliac bones, knees, and elbows;** chronic conjunctivitis, **sclerosing keratitis, and chorioretinal lesions** on eye exam.

Labs CBC/PBS: **eosinophilia.** Fifty-milligram dose of **diethylcarbamazine produces severe pruritus, rash, fever, and conjunctivitis.**

Micro Pathology Skin biopsy at iliac crest shows microfilariae.

PARASITOLOGY

case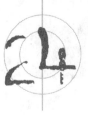

Onchocerciasis

Differential

Hypersensitivity Reaction
Leprosy
Syphilis
Vitamin A Deficiency

Discussion

Onchocerciasis is caused by *Onchocerca volvulus* and is transmitted by the blackfly (*similium* SPECIES), which breeds near rivers; hence it is also known as **river blindness**. Larvae migrate through subcutaneous tissue, producing **painless soft tissue edema** (CALABAR EDEMA); with time, subcutaneous nodules form and filariae obstruct dermal lymphatics, producing atrophy and hypopigmentation. Microfilariae concentrate in the eyes, leading to **chorioretinitis and blindness**.

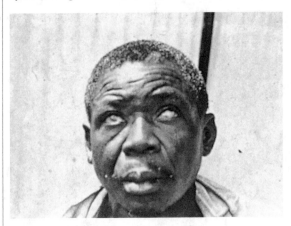

Figure 24-1. A blind patient with onchocerciasis.

Breakout Point

Treatment of patients with **onchocerciasis** with **diethylcarbamazine** results in **massive death of microfilia with eosinophil degradation**. This causes severe **pruritus, rash, fever, and conjunctivitis, the so-called Mazzotti reaction.**

Treatment

Ivermectin; suramin.

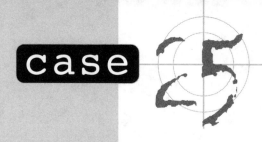
ID/CC   A **4-year-old** boy is brought to the physician by his parents, who complain that the child has had **intense perianal itching,** especially **during the night.**

HPI   The child is otherwise healthy, and his developmental progress is normal.

PE   Perianal excoriation noted.

Labs   Cellulose adhesive tape secured to perianal area during the night reveals presence of **eggs** that were **flattened on one side, were embryonated, and had a thick shell**; no parasites found on stool exam.

PARASITOLOGY

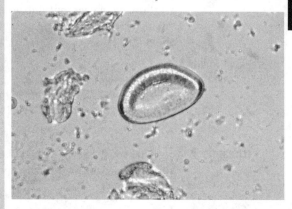

Figure 25-1. Flat-sided embryonated egg retrieved from adhesive tape.

case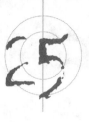

Pinworm Infection

Differential	Proctitis
	Atopic Eczema
	Candidiasis
	Lichen Planus
	Tinea Cruris
Discussion	Infection is caused by *Enterobius vermicularis.* Adult worms are located primarily in the cecal region; **female adult worms migrate to the perianal area during the night and deposit their eggs.** Direct person-to-person **infection occurs by** ingestion and **swallowing of eggs; autoinoculation** occurs by contamination of fingers. The life cycle is completed in about 6 weeks.

Breakout Point

> **Commonly associated with day care facilities, *Enterobius vermicularis* is the most common helminth infection in the United States.**

Treatment	Strict **personal hygiene;** drugs used include **albendazole, mebendazole, piperazine,** and **pyrantel pamoate.**

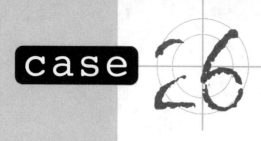

ID/CC An Asian refugee **family** comprising a 30-year-old man, his wife, and 2 schoolchildren present **with complaints of severe itching** over their entire bodies except for their faces; the itching increases **during the night.**

HPI The male family members also report penile and scrotal skin lesions. The family is of **low socioeconomic status** and lives in a single room under **crowded conditions.**

PE Papulovesicular lesions; **"burrows"** seen in the dorsal interdigital web spaces and flexor aspects of both wrists; lesions also seen around elbows, anterior axillary folds, periumbilical area, lower buttocks, and thighs; **face was spared; scrotal and penile lesions** seen in male members were **nodular** and reddish.

PARASITOLOGY

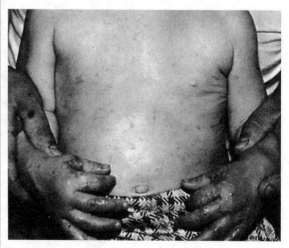

Figure 26-1. Blisters on hands of an infested child.

51

case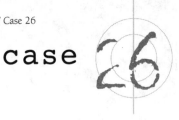

Scabies

Differential

Contact Dermatitis

Folliculitis

Lice

Psoriasis

Urticaria

Chicken Pox

Discussion

Scabies is caused by infestation with ***Sarcoptes scabiei*, a mite** that bores into the corneal layer of the skin, forming burrows in which it deposits its eggs. The scabies organism does not survive for more than 48 hours away from the host; modes of transmission include close contact with infected individuals, unsanitary conditions, and sexual contact. In adults, certain areas of the body are generally spared, including the face, scalp, and neck.

Treatment

Apply **lindane** or **permethrin** (lindane is contraindicated in small children and in pregnant women). All family members must be treated; clothing, linen, and the like should be boiled and washed; fingernails should be trimmed. Use antihistamines or calamine lotion to help control itching and antibiotics if secondary bacterial infection is present. Give ivermectin when topical treatment is impractical.

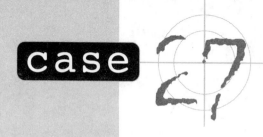

PARASITOLOGY

ID/CC A 27-year-old Peace Corps volunteer working in the **Congo** is sent home after developing **fever, sweats, and abdominal pain** that have not responded to antimalarial treatment.

HPI Five weeks ago, he developed **severe itching and a macular rash** (SWIMMER'S ITCH) after swimming in a nearby pond.

PE VS: fever. PE: moderate enlargement of liver and spleen; tender abdomen but no peritoneal irritation.

Labs CBC/PBS: **marked eosinophilia.** Characteristic large parasite **eggs** with **lateral spines** may be found in stool specimen.

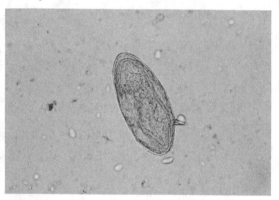

Figure 27-1. Trematode ovum with prominent lateral spine.

Imaging Sigmoidoscopy: swollen and erythematous mucosa; many small ulcerations. CT/US, abdomen: hepatosplenomegaly; portal vein dilatation.

Gross Pathology Skin and liver sites of principal lesions in acute stage; eggs may be found in liver, lungs, intestines, pancreas, spleen, urogenital organs, and brain; chronic stage characterized by **granuloma formation in bladder and liver** (PERIPORTAL FIBROSIS).

Micro Pathology Granulomatous reaction and fibrosis.

53

case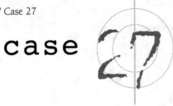

Schistosomiasis

Differential
Leishmaniasis
Malaria
Myeloproliferative Disease
Typhoid Fever
Urethral Cancer

Discussion
Schistosomiasis is among the most common parasitic diseases in the world; infection with *Schistosoma mansoni* or *Schistosoma japonicum* is acquired by **swimming** in **snail-infested ponds** and lakes. Long-standing infection may lead to noncirrhotic portal fibrosis and portal hypertension. Also known as bilharziasis.

Treatment
Praziquantel.

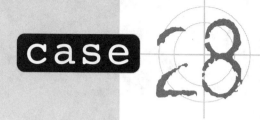

ID/CC A 12-year-old **immigrant from the Middle East** presents with **terminal hematuria**, dysuria, and increased frequency of micturition.

HPI He remembers having played and **bathed in snail-infested streams** while he was in his native country; on one occasion he had developed an **intensely pruritic skin eruption** after bathing in one such stream (CERCARIAL DERMATITIS).

PE Pallor noted.

Labs UA: **hematuria**; mild proteinuria and sterile (**abacterial) pyuria.** Microscopic exam of urine and rectal biopsy reveals presence of **ellipsoid eggs with a sharp terminal spine** containing a miracidium surrounded by a thick, rigid shell.

PARASITOLOGY

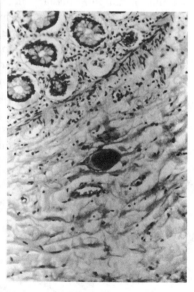

Figure 28-1. Ellipsoid eggs, with a sharp terminal spine, in the bladder wall.

Imaging XR: bladder wall calcification.

case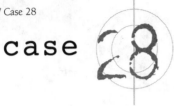

Urinary Schistosomiasis

Differential
: Hemorrhagic Cystitis
Bladder Cancer
Tuberculosis
Amyloidosis

Discussion
: **Three major species** exist. *Schistosoma mansoni,
Schistosoma japonicum*, and *Schistosoma haematobium*
infect humans. *S. mansoni* is found in Africa, the
Arabian Peninsula, South America, and parts of the
Caribbean; *S. japonicum* is found in Japan, China, and
the Philippines; and *S. haematobium* **is found in
Africa and the Middle East.** Transmission of schistosomiasis **cannot occur in the United States**
because of the absence of the specific freshwater **snail
that is an intermediary host.** In *S. haematobium*
infection, the principal symptoms are terminal hematuria, dysuria, and frequent urination; **hydronephro-
sis,** pyelonephritis, and **squamous cell carcinoma of
the urinary bladder** may develop as **complications.**
In *S. mansoni* **and** *S. japonicum* infections, manifestations may include **fever, malaise, abdominal pain,
diarrhea,** or hepatosplenomegaly. Presinusoidal hepatic
trapping of eggs and the consequent granulomatous
reaction induce **portal hypertension.**

Treatment
: **Praziquantel,** metrifonate.

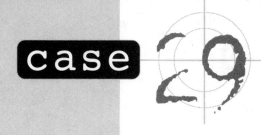
ID/CC A 7-year-old girl is seen by the embassy doctor in **Nigeria** for abdominal pain, **diarrhea, fever, dry cough,** and marked **dyspnea** of 2 weeks' duration.

HPI She is the daughter of an American diplomat working in Nigeria. Despite her parent's admonitions, she frequently **walks barefoot.**

PE VS: fever. PE: moderate respiratory distress; no cyanosis; no clubbing; coarse, crepitant rales and **wheezing** heard over both lung fields; mild abdominal tenderness.

Labs CBC/PBS: **marked eosinophilia.** Typical **motile rhabditiform larvae** on sputum exam as well as in freshly passed stool; positive filarial ELISA and IFA.

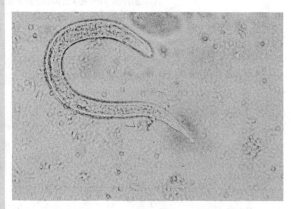

Figure 29-1. Rhabditiform larvae in stool specimen.

Imaging CXR: **bilateral, transient migratory infiltrates.**

Gross Pathology Pneumonitis produced by migration of larvae through respiratory tract.

case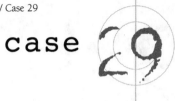

Strongyloidiasis

Differential

Diverticulitis

Eosinophilia

Asthma

Inflammatory Bowel Disease

Malabsorption

Discussion

Strongyloidiasis is seen in the presence of **poor hygiene** and in tropical countries. Larvae penetrate the skin, gaining entrance to the venous system and to the lungs, and then ascend to enter the GI tract. Life-threatening disseminated infection occurs in immunocompromised patients.

Breakout Point

> ***Strongyloides stercoralis*** **is the smallest of the human intestinal nematodes. It is capable of autoinfectious cycles.**

Treatment

Ivermectin, thiabendazole.

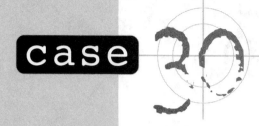
PARASITOLOGY

ID/CC A 40-year-old man who recently went **hiking in a forest** in the **western United States** presents with **symmetric weakness** of the lower extremities that has now progressed over the past few days to involve the trunk and the upper arms.

HPI The patient does not report any sensory symptoms.

PE Higher mental functions intact; **symmetric flaccid paralysis** with an **ascending pattern** of spread noted; **no sensory loss** demonstrated; on careful examination of hairy areas of the body, a **tick** was found **embedded in the scalp.**

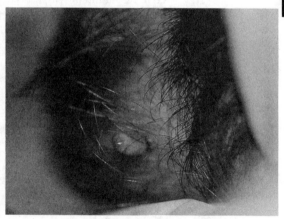

Figure 30-1. Engorged tick in hairline.

Labs LP: CSF normal. EMG: nerve conduction velocity and compound muscle action potentials decreased.

case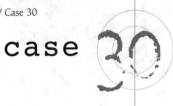

Tick Paralysis

Differential
Bell Palsy
Herpes Zoster
Botulism
Multiple Sclerosis

Discussion
Feeding ticks may elaborate a **neurotoxin** that causes tick paralysis; symmetric weakness of the lower extremities progresses to an **ascending flaccid paralysis** over several hours to days, although the sensorium remains clear and sensory function is normal.

Treatment
Tick was detached without being squeezed, and this led to resolution of symptoms over the next few days.

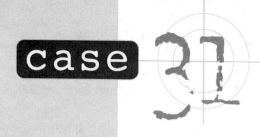
case 31

ID/CC	A 40-year-old man diagnosed with **AIDS** presents with a **severe headache**.
HPI	He suffered a grand mal seizure 2 hours before his arrival in the ER. He denies any history of seizures and adds that he has many pets, including **cats**.
PE	**Generalized lymphadenopathy;** bilateral **papilledema;** left-sided hemiparesis with hyperactive deep tendon reflexes on left side; positive Babinski sign on left side.
Labs	Positive indirect fluorescent antibody test for toxoplasmosis; positive Sabin-Feldman dye test.
Imaging	MR/CT, head: single rounded **mass lesions with ring or nodular enhancement.**

PARASITOLOGY

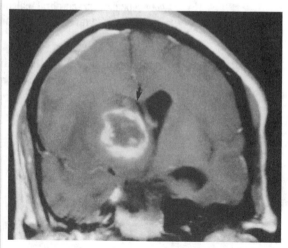

Figure 31-1. Coronal MR imaging of a solitary ring enhancing intracranial lesion.

case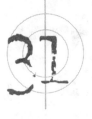

Toxoplasmosis

Differential

Brain Abscess
Lymphoma
Tuberculosis
Metastatic Cancer
Sarcoidosis
Primary CNS Neoplasm

Discussion

The **definitive host** of *Toxoplasma gondii* is the domestic cat. The intermediate hosts are many and varied, including humans. Toxoplasmosis is also transmitted by ingestion of raw or undercooked meat and vertically from infected mothers to the fetus.

Breakout Point

> **Toxoplasmosis** can **cross the placenta** and cause congenital toxoplasmosis characterized by microcephaly, **intracerebral calcifications, chorioretinitis,** and **mental retardation.**

Treatment

Pyrimethamine and **sulfadiazine** in combination; add leucovorin to prevent bone marrow suppression.

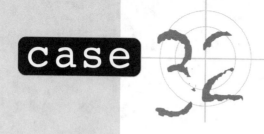

ID/CC	A 50-year-old man presents with generalized **myalgia** and a persistent **low-grade fever**.
HPI	In addition, the patient recalled having severe **abdominal pain and diarrhea several weeks ago.** The patient worked in a **pig slaughterhouse** for many years.
PE	VS: fever. PE: periorbital and facial edema; tenderness over calf, thigh, and shoulder muscles; conjunctival and splinter hemorrhages; no neurologic deficit seen.
Labs	CBC: **eosinophilia.** Normal ESR; **elevated serum CPK, LDH, and AST.**
Gross Pathology	Facial, neck, biceps, lower back, and diaphragm most frequently affected muscles.
Micro Pathology	Biopsy of sternocleidomastoid muscle reveals larval cysts in muscle.

PARASITOLOGY

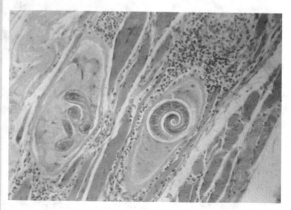

Figure 32-1. Encapsulated larvae within skeletal muscle.

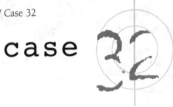

case 32

Trichinosis

Differential	Angioedema
	Food Poisoning
	Gastroenteritis
	Polyarteritis Nodosa
	Influenza
	Typhoid Fever
Discussion	The organism causing trichinosis, *Trichinella spiralis*, can be transmitted when **raw or undercooked pork** is ingested. The larvae develop only in **striated muscle cells.**

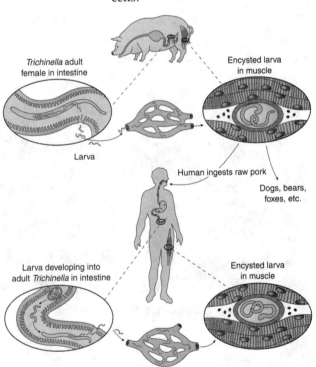

Figure 32-2. *Trichinella spiralis* infection cycle.

Treatment	Albendazole; mebendazole; high-dose corticosteroids.

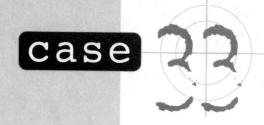

case 33

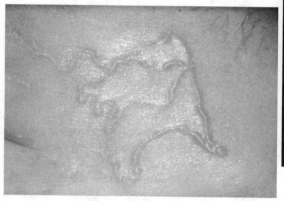

PARASITOLOGY

ID/CC An 8-year-old boy is brought to a physician with complaints of **serpiginous urticarial skin rashes on the face,** and ill-defined muscle aches.

Figure 33-1. Serpiginous urticarial skin rashes on the face.

HPI The child's mother has caught the child eating dirt or soil on many occasions (PICA). The family also has a **pet dog** at home.

PE **Rounded swelling near the optic disk** seen on fundus exam of left eye; **urticarial wheals** observed on extremities and trunk; mild **hepatosplenomegaly** noted.

Labs Leukocytosis with marked **eosinophilia;** EIA using extracts of excretory-secretory products of *Ancylostoma braziliense* larvae is positive.

Micro Pathology Biopsy of liver reveals larvae with granuloma and eosinophilic infiltration.

case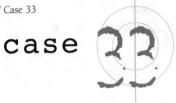

Cutaneous Larva Migrans

Differential

Hypersensitivity Pneumonitis

Löffler Syndrome

Tinea Infection

Urticaria

Vasculitis

Atopic Skin Disease

Discussion

When the nondefinitive human host is infected with parasites that normally infect animals, the parasites do not mature completely, but the larvae introduced persist and induce an inflammatory reaction. The syndrome of **visceral larva migrans** develops when nematode larvae of animal parasites (**mostly cat or dog ascarids** such as *Toxocara canis*) migrate in human tissues; the syndrome of **cutaneous larva migrans** (creeping eruption) develops when the larvae of various parasites (including the **dog or cat hookworm** *Ancylostoma braziliense*) penetrate human skin and form pruritic, serpiginous cutaneous lesions along the migratory tracts of the larvae.

Treatment

Diethylcarbamazine; albendazole or **mebendazole;** steroids to control symptomatic inflammatory response; laser photocoagulation of visible ocular larvae.

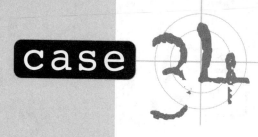

case 34

ID/CC A 7-year-old boy is brought to his family physician complaining of a **thick yellowish discharge in his eyes that prevents him from opening his eyes in the morning**; for the past few days, his eyes have been **blood red, painful**, and **watery**. His eye pain is exacerbated by exposure to light (PHOTOPHOBIA).

HPI Three of his classmates and a neighbor had a similar episode about 7 days ago (suggesting a **local epidemic** of such cases).

PE VS: no fever. PE: **normal visual acuity; erythematous palpebral conjunctiva**; watery eyes; **remains of thick mucus** found on inner canthal area; no corneal infiltrate on slit-lamp exam; normal anterior chamber; **mild preauricular lymphadenopathy.**

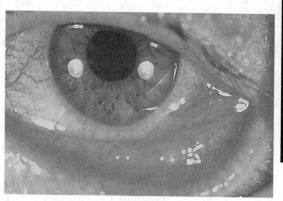

Figure 34-1. Watery conjunctival discharge and conjunctival hyperemia. The lower lid is retracted inferiorly, demonstrating tarsal conjunctival edema and injection.

Labs Stained conjunctival smears reveal **lymphocytes**, giant cells, **neutrophils**, and bacteria.

case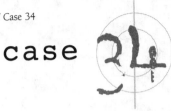

Acute Conjunctivitis

Differential	Corneal Abrasion
	Glaucoma
	Herpes Zoster
	Scleritis
	Iritises
	Uveitis
Discussion	Conjunctivitis is a common disease of childhood that is mostly viral **(adenovirus)** and self-limiting; it occurs in epidemics, and secondary bacterial infections (staphylococci and streptococci) may result. Visual acuity is not affected.
Treatment	Topical antimicrobial eye drops; cool compresses; minimize contact with others to avoid spread; avoid use of topical steroid preparations, as these can exacerbate bacterial and viral eye infections.

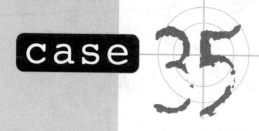
ID/CC A 28-year-old **homosexual man** complains of continuous low-grade **fever, weight loss,** and **diarrhea** of 1 month's duration.

HPI He also complains of an **extensive skin rash, mucous membrane eruptions, recurrent herpes zoster infection,** and **oral ulcerations.** He reports practicing receptive anal intercourse.

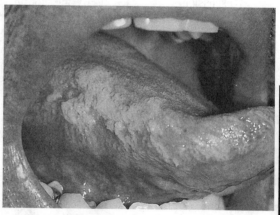

Figure 35-1. Oral leukoplakia.

PE VS: low-grade fever. PS: cachectic; **generalized lymphadenopathy;** maculopapular rash; severe **seborrheic dermatitis; aphthous ulcers;** white confluent patch with corrugated surface along lateral borders of tongue; **penile warts;** extensive multiple pruritic, pink, umbilicated papules 2 to 5 mm in diameter.

Labs CBC: anemia; leukopenia with lymphopenia; thrombocytopenia. **Low CD4 count** (200–500); elevated CD8 T-cell count.

Micro Pathology **Oral hairy leukoplakia;** lesions show keratin projections resembling hairs, koilocytosis, and little atypia; hybridization techniques reveal **EBV** in lesions.

VIROLOGY

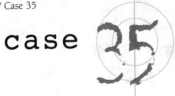

case

Acquired Immunodeficiency Syndrome–Related Complex

Differential

Immunosuppression
CMV Infection
Diabetes
Bacillary Angiomatosis
Tuberculosis
Overwhelming Fungal Infection

Discussion

The stage of HIV infection in which CD4 counts are <200 µL has been given a variety of names, including ARC. Diseases manifested during this stage are not sufficiently indicative of a defect in cell-mediated immunity to be considered AIDS-defining illnesses.

Breakout Point

> **Testing in HIV/AIDS**
>
> **ELISA** for HIV-1 **screening**; if positive, then **Western blot for confirmation**; **PCR** for viral RNA copy number to monitor therapy.

■ TABLE 35-1 AIDS-DEFINING OPPORTUNISTIC INFECTIONS IN HIV-INFECTED PATIENTS

- Candidiasis of the trachea, bronchi, or lungs
- Esophageal candidiasis
- Disseminated coccidiodomycosis
- Extrapulmonary cryptococcosis
- Chronic cryptosporidiosis, with diarrhea for more than 1 month
- CMV infection (other than liver, spleen, or nodes)
- CMV retinitis (with vision loss)
- HIV encephalopathy
- Herpes simplex: chronic ulcers for more than 1 month, or bronchitis, pneumonia, or esophagitis.
- Disseminated or extrapulmonary histoplasmosis
- Isoporiasis, with diarrhea for more than 1 month
- Kaposi sarcoma
- Non-Hodgkin lymphoma of B cell or unknown phenotype, including Burkitt lymphoma

- Primary lymphoma of the brain
- Disseminated *Mycobacterium avium* complex or *M. kansasii*
- *Mycobacterium tuberculosis,* either pulmonary or extrapulmonary
- Other disseminated or extrapulmonary mycobacterial infections
- *Pneumocystis jiroveci* pneumonia
- Progressive multifocal leukoencephalopathy
- Recurrent *Salmonella* septicemia
- Toxoplasmosis of the brain
- Wasting syndrome caused by HIV
- Invasive cervical cancer

Treatment

Prophylactic antibiotics for prevention of opportunistic infections while monitoring CD4 T-cell counts; antiretroviral drugs (zidovudine, didanosine, zalcitabine, and protease inhibitors); counseling and rehabilitative measures.

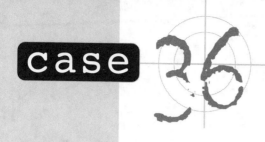

case 36

ID/CC An **8-year-old child** with **sickle-cell anemia** is seen with complaints of sudden-onset **pallor of the skin** and mucous membranes, fatigue, and malaise.

HPI The child suffered a **mild prodromal illness** before developing severe pallor.

PE VS: no fever; tachycardia; tachypnea; BP normal. PE: severe pallor; mild icterus; no lymphadenopathy, splenomegaly, or hepatomegaly noted.

Labs CBC: **severe anemia** (Hb 2 g/dL); **reduced leukocyte** and platelet counts; mild hyperbilirubinemia; **absent reticulocytes** and sickled RBCs on peripheral blood smear.

Micro Pathology Bone marrow biopsy reveals increased numbers of **giant pronormoblasts**.

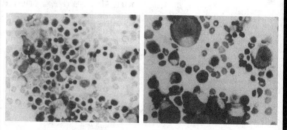

Figure 36-1. Cytopathic giant pronormoblasts in bone marrow.

VIROLOGY

case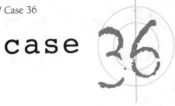

Anemia—Aplastic Crisis (Parvovirus 19)

Differential

Rubella
Scarlet Fever
Drug Eruption
Collagen Vascular Disease

Discussion

Parvovirus infection is the cause of **transient aplastic crises** (may also be due to folic acid deficiency) that occur in patients who have severe **hemolytic disorders**; cessation of erythropoiesis for about 10 days in a normal adult as a result of parvovirus infection would produce a 10% drop in hemoglobin concentration (i.e., a fall of 1% daily would lead to a decline in hemoglobin concentration of 1 to 2 g/dL after 10 days). A patient with severe hemolysis in whom the bone marrow is turning over at a rate 7 times normal would experience a 70% decrease in hemoglobin concentration (i.e., a drop from 10 g/dL to 3 g/dL) as a result of a 10-day cessation of erythropoiesis. Although parvovirus can affect all precursor cells, the red cell precursors are most profoundly affected.

Treatment

Blood transfusions to tide over the crisis. Spontaneous recovery in 1 to 2 weeks.

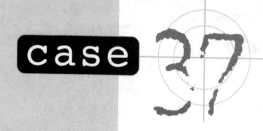
ID/CC	A 13-year-old White girl visits her pediatrician complaining of **fever**, severe **dyspnea**, and a **dry cough**.
HPI	She was recently diagnosed with acute lymphocytic leukemia, for which she received a **bone marrow** transplant. She is currently on **immunosuppressive therapy**.
PE	VS: fever; **tachypnea**. PE: pallor; **crepitant rales** over both lung fields; mild cyanosis; no hepatosplenomegaly.
Labs	CBC/PBS: anemia; leukopenia. ABGs: **hypoxemia**. No organism in induced sputum stained with Gram, Giemsa, ZN, and methenamine silver.
Imaging	CXR: diffuse, bilateral interstitial infiltrates.
Gross Pathology	**Interstitial pneumonitis**; hepatitis.
Micro Pathology	Characteristic **intranuclear inclusions with surrounding halo** (OWL'S- OR BULL'S-EYE CELLS) on transbronchial lung biopsy.

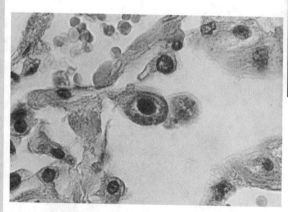

Figure 37-1. Intranuclear inclusion body (giving the appearance of an owl's eye).

VIROLOGY

case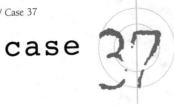

Cytomegalovirus Pneumonitis

Differential | Adenovirus
Influenza
Bacterial Pneumonia
Parainfluenza virus
Fungal Pneumonia
Varicella-Zoster Virus

Discussion | An enveloped, dsDNA virus belonging to the herpesvirus group, it is the most common cause of pneumonia and death in **bone marrow transplant patients.** It is also common in **patients who have AIDS.**

Treatment | **Ganciclovir** or foscarnet.

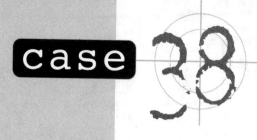
ID/CC A 30-year-old homosexual White man presents to his family physician with a **rapidly progressive diminution of vision.**

HPI He is known to be **HIV positive** and periodically comes in for checkups.

PE **Cotton-wool exudates, necrotizing retinitis, and perivascular hemorrhages** on funduscopic exam.

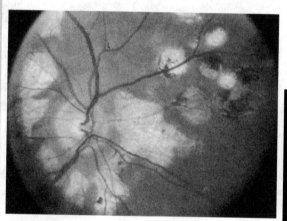

Figure 38-1. Patchy, yellow-white lesions known as cotton-wool spots.

VIROLOGY

75

case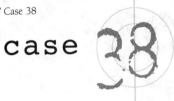

Cytomegalovirus Retinitis

Differential
HIV Infection
Herpes Zoster
Toxoplasmosis
Lymphocytic Choriomengitis Virus
Rubella
Enteroviral Infection

Discussion
CMV retinitis is an important **treatable cause of blindness** that occurs in 20% of patients with AIDS; 50% to 60% of patients develop retinal detachment within 1 year. **Toxoplasmosis** and **PML** are other important causes of blindness in patients infected with AIDS.

Treatment
Ganciclovir; foscarnet; cidofovir.

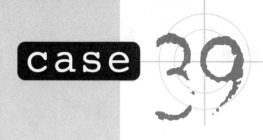

case 39

ID/CC A newborn baby is referred to the pediatrician for further evaluation of an US **small head,** low birth weight, and an extensive **erythematous rash.**

HPI **Intrauterine growth retardation** was prenatally diagnosed on US. The child's **mother had a flulike** episode during the **first trimester** of her pregnancy.

PE Small for gestational age; generalized hypotonia with sluggish neonatal reflexes; extensive **"pinpoint" petechial skin rash** (MULBERRY MUFFIN RASH); **microcephaly; chorioretinitis;** mild **icterus; hepatosplenomegaly; sensorineural hearing loss** in right ear.

Labs CBC/PBS: mild thrombocytopenia; atypical lymphocytosis. Moderately elevated direct serum bilirubin and transaminases; shell vial cultures positive for CMV. UA: cells in urine found to have large **intranuclear inclusions.**

Imaging XR/CT, head: **periventricular calcifications; microcephaly.**

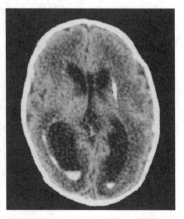

Figure 39-1. Unenhanced head CT of an infant, showing a dense periventricular calcification as well as an intraventricular hemorrhage.

VIROLOGY

case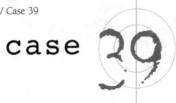

Cytomegalovirus—Congenital

Differential

HIV Infection
Herpes Zoster
Toxoplasmosis
Lymphocytic Choriomengitis Virus
Rubella
Enteroviral Infection

Discussion

A congenital herpesvirus infection involving the CNS, with eye and ear damage, congenital CMV is a common cause of mental retardation.

Breakout Point

> **Cytomegalovirus** is one of the **TORCH complex** members of congenital infectious agents leading **to multiple malformations.**
> TORCH includes: *T*oxoplasmosis, *O*thers (HIV, syphilis, etc.), *R*ubella, *C*MV, *H*erpes

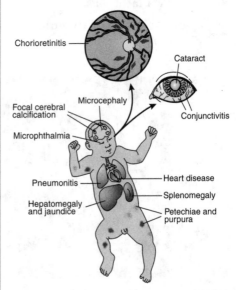

Figure 39-2. Consequences of congenital CMV infection.

Treatment

Ganciclovir may slow progression of sensorineural deafness; neurodevelopmental monitoring and therapy.

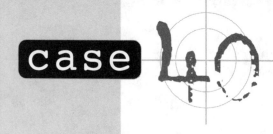

case 40

ID/CC A 28-year-old man who lives in the **northwestern United States** complains of a high-grade **fever with rigors,** generalized aches, myalgias, headache, and backache.

HPI Four days ago he returned from a hiking trip during which he was **bitten by a tick;** he took amoxicillin as prophylaxis against Lyme disease.

PE VS: fever.

Labs CBC: leukopenia; relative lymphocytosis. Viral antigen detected in RBCs by immunofluorescence.

case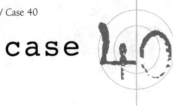

Colorado Tick Fever

Differential

Ehrlichiosis
Lyme Disease
Q Fever
Rocky Mountain Spotted Fever
Tularemia

Discussion

Colorado tick fever virus is an 80-nm, double-shelled, **reovirus** that is covered with capsomeres; its icosahedral core contains **12 segments of dsRNA**. The disease is a zoonosis that is transmitted by a wood tick, *Dermacentor andersoni*. It occurs primarily in the U.S. Rocky Mountain region, primarily affecting hikers. Since no specific therapy exists, prevention is key (wear clothing that covers the body).

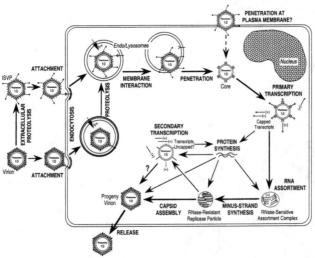

Figure 40-1. The life cycle of a reovirus.

Breakout Point

Segmented RNA Viruses
• Bunyavirus
• Orthomyxovirus
• Reovirus

Treatment

Symptomatic.

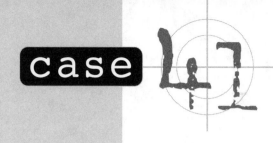

case 47

ID/CC	A 20-year-old man presents with a **runny nose, nasal congestion, sore throat, headache, and sneezing.**
HPI	He notes that his wife currently has similar symptoms.
PE	VS: mild fever. PE: rhinorrhea; congested and inflamed posterior pharyngeal wall; no lymphadenopathy.
Labs	Routine tests normal; routine throat swab staining and culture negative for bacteria.
Gross Pathology	Nasal membranes **edematous and erythematous** with watery discharge.
Micro Pathology	Mononuclear inflammation of mucosa; focal desquamation.

VIROLOGY

case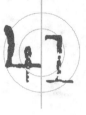

Common Cold (Viral)

Differential
Adenovirus Infection
Bronchitis
Coxsackie Virus Infection
Influenza
Parainfluenza
Coronavirus Infection
Respiratory Syncytial Virus Infection

Discussion
Colds occur 2 to 3 times a year in the average person in the United States; the peak incidence is in the winter months. **Rhinoviruses** account for the majority of viral URIs, followed by coronaviruses. Spread occurs by **direct contact** and respiratory droplets.

■ **TABLE 41-1 COMMON CAUSES OF THE COLD AND SEASONAL VARIATIONS**

Virus	Percentage of Common Cold	Usual Season
Rhinovirus	15–40	Early autumn and early spring
Respiratory syncytial virus	25 in children	Late autumn through spring
Coronavirus	10–20	Late autumn through early spring
Parainfluenza	5	Spring
Adenovirus	>2	Autumn through spring
Coxsackie virus	9	Summer and early fall

Treatment
Symptomatic.

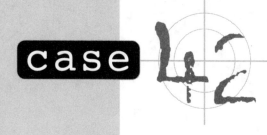

ID/CC A **2-year-old** toddler is brought to the ER by his parents with **sore throat, inspiratory stridor,** and a barking cough of 1 day's duration.

HPI The patient has no significant past medical history.

PE VS: fever (38.6°C); tachypnea. PE: **respiratory distress;** nasopharyngeal discharge; diffuse rhonchi and wheezes; examination of extremities reveals some cyanosis.

Labs Throat and nasal swabs isolate **parainfluenza virus;** serodiagnosis and hemagglutinin inhibition tests reveal type 1 (most common cause).

Imaging CXR: air trapping. XR, neck: **subglottic narrowing.** Characteristic **Steeple sign.**

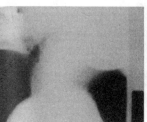 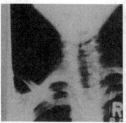

Figure 42-1. Lateral **(left)** and anteroposterior **(right)** soft-tissue radiographs of the child. Note the characteristic Steeple sign in the anteroposterior radiograph.

VIROLOGY

Gross Pathology Inflammation and edema of larynx, trachea, and bronchi.

case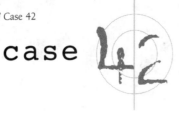

Croup

Differential | Diphtheria
Epiglottitis
Inhalation Injury
Bacterial Tracheitis
Retropharyngeal Abscess

Discussion | Differentiate croup from *Haemophilus influenzae* type B and influenza A virus. Modes of transmission include respiratory droplets and person-to-person contact; tends to peak in the fall and winter. Most cases of croup are due to parainfluenza virus type 1; type 3 is a prominent cause of bronchiolitis in babies.

■ TABLE 42-1 COMPARISON OF EPIGLOTTIS AND CROUP

	Epiglottis	Croup
Anatomy	Supraglottic	Subglottic
Etiology	Bacterial: *Haemophilus influenza*	Viral: Parainfluenza
Age range	3–7 yrs, adults	0.5–3
Onset	6–24 hrs	24–72
Toxicity	Marked	Mild to moderate
Drooling	Frequent	Absent
Cough	Unusual	Frequent
Hoarseness	Unusual	Frequent
Webs	Leukocytes	Normal

Treatment | Most cases respond to **supportive therapy** such as humidified air, removal of secretions, and bed rest. Severe cases may require humidified oxygen, racemic epinephrine, or high-dose corticosteroids.

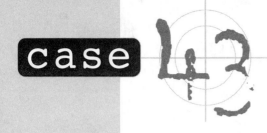
ID/CC   A **10-year-old** boy complains of a spreading **skin rash** and **painful** swelling of both **wrists.**

HPI   The patient's mother states that the rash began with **erythema of the cheeks** (SLAPPED-CHEEK APPEARANCE) and subsequently progressed to involve the trunk and limbs.

PE   **Erythematous lacy/reticular skin rash** involving face, trunk, and limbs; bilateral swelling and painful restriction of movement at both **wrist joints.**

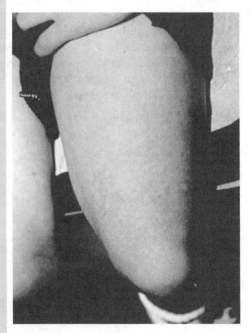

Figure 43-1. A lacy reticular pattern of erythema on the involved thigh.

Labs   Serology detects presence of **specific IgM antibody to parvovirus;** ASO titer (to rule out acute rheumatic fever) normal; rheumatoid factor (to rule out rheumatoid arthritis) negative.

VIROLOGY

case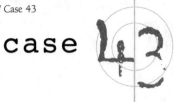

Erythema Infectiosum

Differential

Measles
Mumps
Roseola Infantum
Scarlet Fever
Hand-Foot-and-Mouth Disease
Drug rash
Allergic Rash

Discussion

A small (20-nm to 26-nm), **single-stranded DNA virus, parvovirus B19** causes erythema infectiosum (fifth disease) in schoolchildren, **aplastic crises** in persons with underlying hemolytic disorders (e.g., sickle-cell anemia), **chronic anemia** in immunocompromised hosts, arthralgia/arthritis in normal individuals, and **fetal loss** in pregnant women.

Treatment

Self-limiting disease.

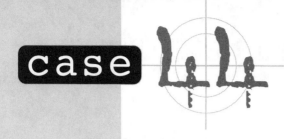

case 44

ID/CC A 25-year-old man presented with sudden-onset **breathlessness, cough, cyanosis, and high-grade fever.**

HPI The patient failed to improve on 100% oxygen, became hypotensive, and **died of type 2 respiratory failure** a few hours after admission. He had been in perfect health and had been **hiking in several rodent-infested areas** before falling ill.

PE On admission he was found to have fever, tachycardia, **cyanosis,** hypotension, and **rales on auscultation** over both lung fields; no meningeal signs or localizing CNS signs could be demonstrated.

Labs ABGs: respiratory acidosis with **hypoxia and hypercapnia.** CBC: leukocytosis; **hemoconcentration; thrombocytopenia;** atypical lymphocytosis. Increased LDH and ALT levels; prolonged PT index; sputum exam and blood culture did not yield any organism.

Imaging CXR: **noncardiogenic pulmonary edema** (bat-wing edema pattern).

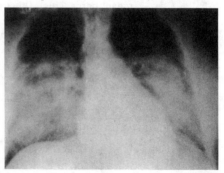

Figure 44-1. Chest radiograph taken 48 hours after admission, showing bilateral interstitial infiltrates (bat wings).

Micro Pathology Histopathologic exam of lung tissues was suggestive of **ARDS** (adult hyaline membrane disease).

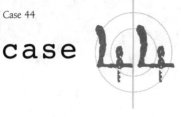

case

Hantaan Pulmonary Syndrome

Differential

ARDS
CHF
Pneumonic Plague
Drug-induced Pulmonary Edema
Bioterrorism
Pneumonia

Discussion

A virus closely related to the **Hantaan virus** (which produces Korean hemorrhagic fever and hemorrhagic fever with renal syndrome) has been recovered from mice in various regions of the United States; **rodents are the natural host** for this group of viruses. Infected rodents shed the virus in saliva, urine, and feces for many weeks, and **humans** are believed to **acquire the infection via exposure to rodent excrement or saliva,** either by the aerosol route or by direct inoculation.

Breakout Point

> Hantaan virus is an example of a **robovirus** (rodent-borne virus), Other roboviruses include members of the bunyaviruses, phleboviruses, and nairoviruses (i.e., Crimean-Congo hemorrhagic fever virus).

Treatment

Intensive ventilatory support; ribavirin; poor prognosis.

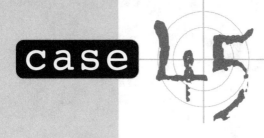
ID/CC   A 10-year-old boy is brought to the ER in a state of **shock** accompanied by **massive hematemesis.**

HPI   The family had just returned from a vacation in **Thailand.** His parents say that he had a high-grade fever for 5 to 6 days, for which he was receiving presumptive treatment for malaria.

PE   VS: hypotension; tachycardia. VS: cool, clammy extremities; **ecchyomotic skin rash** over extremities, axillae, trunk, and face; bleeding from venipuncture sites.

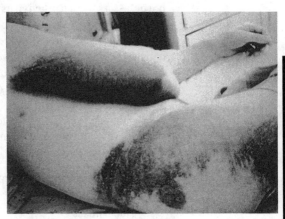

Figure 45-1. Extensive ecchymoses.

Labs   CBC: **thrombocytopenia; hematocrit increased** by >20%. Abnormal clotting profile suggestive of **DIC.**

Imaging   US: bilateral pleural effusion and ascites.

VIROLOGY

case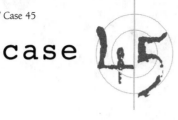

Hemorrhagic Fever—Dengue

Differential

Malaria
Yellow Fever
Typhoid
Leptospirosis
West Nile Virus
Crimean Congo Fever
Ebola Virus

Discussion

Dengue hemorrhagic fever is caused by a **mosquito-borne** (*Aedes aegypti*) **flavivirus** and is characterized by four distinct dengue serotypes (type 2 is considered the most dangerous). *A. aegypti* has a domestic habitat (stagnant water in flower pots, old jars, tin cans, and old tires) and bites during the day. Dengue fever has shown an increase in incidence in **Southeast Asia, Central and South America**, and the **Caribbean**. Since no specific therapy exists, prevent by avoiding contact with infected *A. aegypti*.

Breakout Point

Arboviruses (Arthropod-borne Viruses) Include Members of
• **Togaviruses**
• **Flaviviruses**
• **Reoviruses**
• **Bunyaviruses**

Treatment

Symptomatic; manage shock with fluids and hemodynamic monitoring; fresh blood/platelet-rich plasma; avoid salicylates.

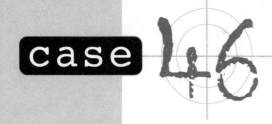

case 46

ID/CC   A 58-year-old man who was hitchhiking through **central and southern Africa** was admitted to a hospital in Zaire in a state of shock following **massive hemorrhage from the GI tract** (hematemesis and melena); he died within 6 hours of admission. Ten days later, a male **doctor who had attended** this patient and had attempted resuscitation became **ill with a similar disease** syndrome.

HPI   At admission, he gave an 8-day history of progressive **fever, severe headaches, myalgias, and watery diarrhea.** He also reported an erythematous, **measles-like skin rash** that had begun to desquamate.

PE   VS: fever. PE: splenomegaly; hepatomegaly.

Labs   CBC: leukopenia; Pelger-Huët anomaly of neutrophils with atypical mononuclear cells; **thrombocytopenia with abnormal platelet aggregation.**

Gross Pathology   At autopsy, **lymph nodes, liver, and spleen** found to be most conspicuously involved.

Micro Pathology   Severe congestion and stasis of spleen; **widespread necrosis** of liver cells; **electron microscopy** of liver revealed **pleomorphic virus particles** appearing in contrast preparations as **long, filamentous forms, U-shaped forms, and some circular forms resembling a doughnut.**

VIROLOGY

case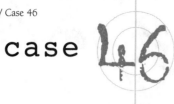

Hemorrhagic Fever—Ebola

Differential

Typhoid Fever
Yellow Fever
Dengue Fever
Crimean Congo Fever
Marburg Virus

Discussion

A hemorrhagic, febrile infection of humans due to infection with the **Ebola** and **Marburg** viruses, both of which are filoviruses that are structurally indistinguishable but antigenically distinct. This disease is a zoonosis but the reservoir is unknown. Individuals can become infected through person-to-person or nosocomial contact.

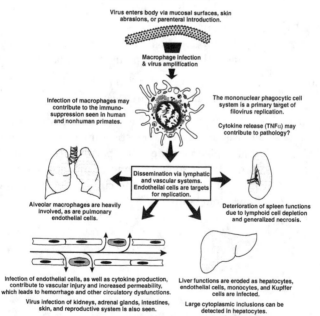

Figure 46-1. Schematic illustration of the events and pathology associated with severe filovirus infections of humans.

Treatment

Supportive care, since no specific treatment exists; outbreak control measures such as isolation and quarantine.

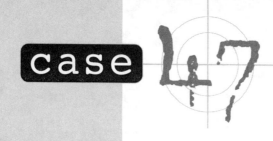

case 47

ID/CC   An 11-year-old White boy presents with **jaundice** and **dark yellow urine** that has been present for the last several days.

HPI   He also complains of nausea, vomiting, and malaise. For the past 2 weeks, he has had a low-grade fever and mild abdominal pain. He recently returned from a **vacation in Mexico,** where he said he consumed a lot of **shellfish.**

PE   Icterus; tender, firm hepatomegaly; no evidence of splenomegaly or free fluid in the peritoneal cavity.

Labs   **Direct hyperbilirubinemia;** elevated serum transaminases (ALT > AST); moderately elevated alkaline phosphatase; prolonged PT; increased urinary urobilinogen and bilirubin.

Gross Pathology   May often appear normal.

Micro Pathology   Multifocal hepatocellular necrosis with Councilman bodies; lymphocytic infiltrates around necrotic foci; loss of lobular architecture.

VIROLOGY

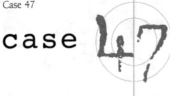

case 47

Hepatitis A

Differential

Budd-Chiari Syndrome
CMV
Drug-induced Liver Damage
Acute HIV Infection
EBV

Discussion

In hepatitis A infection, virus is shed 14 to 21 days before the onset of **jaundice;** patients are no longer infectious 7 days after the onset of jaundice. It is spread by **fecal-oral transmission** and is endemic in areas where there are **contaminated water sources.** There is **no chronic carrier state;** recovery takes place in 6 to 12 months. HAV is a naked, single-stranded RNA virus of the **picorna** family. A killed vaccine is available; passive immunization in the form of immune serum globulins is also available.

Breakout Point

Medically Important Single-stranded (+) Genome RNA Viruses
• Picornavirus
• Calicivirus
• Flavivirus
• Togovirus
• Retrovirus
• Coronavirus

Treatment

Supportive management; passive vaccination available.

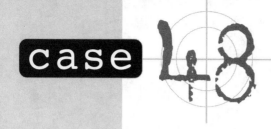
ID/CC A 25-year-old man who is a medical student presents with **jaundice** and **dark yellow urine.**

HPI He admits to having experienced an accidental **needle stick** 2 months ago, which he did not report. He also complains of nausea, low-grade fever, and loss of appetite.

PE Icterus; tender, firm **hepatomegaly;** no evidence of ascites or splenomegaly.

Labs **Direct hyperbilirubinemia;** elevated serum transaminases (ALT > AST); mildly elevated alkaline phosphatase; **serology pending.**

Imaging US, abdomen: hepatomegaly; increased echogenicity.

Gross Pathology Liver may be enlarged, congested, or jaundiced; in fulminant cases of massive hepatic necrosis, liver becomes small, shrunken, and soft (acute yellow atrophy).

Micro Pathology Liver biopsy reveals hepatocellular necrosis with **Councilman bodies** and ballooning degeneration; inflammation of portal areas with infiltration of mononuclear cells (small lymphocytes, plasma cells, eosinophils); prominence of Kupffer cells and bile ducts; cholestasis with bile plugs.

VIROLOGY

case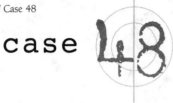

Hepatitis B—Acute

Differential | Alcoholic Hepatitis
Autoimmune Hepatitis
Hemochromatosis
Hepatocellular Carcinoma
Hepatitis A
Wilson Disease

Discussion | **Hepatitis B immune globulin** plus **hepatitis B vaccine** are recommended for parenteral or mucosal exposure to blood and for newborns of HBsAg-positive mothers. The infection is divided into the prodromal, icteric, and convalescent phases; **5% proceed to chronic hepatitis** with increased risk for cirrhosis and **hepatocellular carcinoma.** Unlike hepatitis A, hepatitis B has a long incubation period (3 months). HBV is an enveloped, partially circular DNA virus of the **hepadna** family that contains a DNA-dependent DNA polymerase. The continued presence of HBsAg after infection has clinically resolved indicates a chronic carrier state.

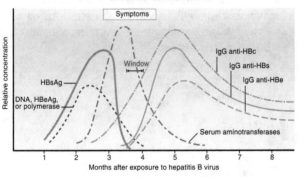

Figure 48-1. Typical course of acute hepatitis B infection.

Treatment | Supportive care; follow up to determine continued presence of HBsAg for at least 6 months as sign of chronic hepatitis; vaccine available for prevention.

Breakout Point |

> The HBV vaccine consists of **recombinant HBsAg** produced in yeast cells.

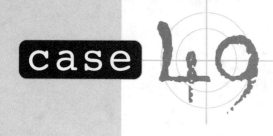
ID/CC A 30-year-old man is referred for an evaluation of **intermittent jaundice** over the past 2 years.

HPI He also complains of diarrhea, skin rash, and weight loss. He received a **blood transfusion** 3 years ago, when he was injured in a motorcycle accident. He denies any IV drug use or any history of neuropsychiatric disorders in his family.

PE **Icterus;** firm, **tender hepatomegaly;** splenomegaly; no evidence of ascites; no Kayser–Fleischer rings found on slit-lamp examination.

Labs Direct hyperbilirubinemia; markedly raised serum transaminase levels; **HBV serology negative.**

Micro Pathology On liver biopsy, presence of ballooning degeneration; fatty changes; **portal inflammation with necrosis of hepatocytes within parenchyma** or immediately adjacent to portal areas (PIECEMEAL NECROSIS).

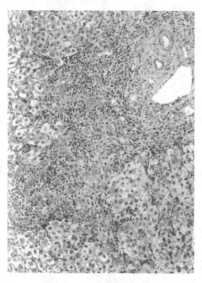

Figure 49-1. Piecemeal necrosis of the periportal parenchyma.

VIROLOGY

97

case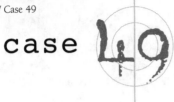

Hepatitis C—Chronic Active

Differential
Autoimmune Hepatitis
Drug-induced Hepatitis
Hemochromatosis
Chronic Hepatitis B
Cholangitis
Wilson Disease

Discussion
Hepatitis C belongs to the **flavivirus** family and is currently the most important cause of **post transfusion viral hepatitis**; 90% of cases involve percutaneous transmission. More than 50% of cases progress to chronic hepatitis, leading to cirrhosis in 20%.

Breakout Point

> HCV is more likely than HBV to cause cirrhosis and hepatocellular carcinoma, however HBV is more common worldwide.

Treatment
Ribavirin and α_{2b}-interferon; supportive management.

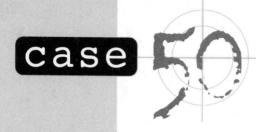

ID/CC A **7-year-old** boy complains of a **high fever** and a very **sore throat**.

HPI The pain is so severe that the child refuses to swallow. He is adequately immunized and achieved normal developmental milestones.

PE VS: fever. PE: **characteristic grayish-white vesicular lesions,** some of which have ulcerated, noted over **soft palate** and **tonsils.**

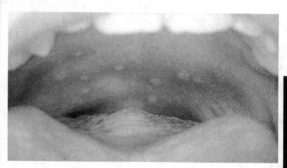

Figure 50-1. Typical pharyngeal lesions.

Labs **Coxsackievirus A** isolated from mucosal lesions.

VIROLOGY

case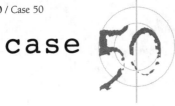

Herpangina

Differential

Coxsackie Infection
Enterovirus Infection
HFMD
Herpes Simplex
Bacterial Pharyngitis

Discussion

In **HFMD**, patients complain of fever, weakness, and decreased appetite along with similar lesions noted in the oral cavity, palms, soles, and buttocks. Herpangina may be caused by coxsackievirus A1–A10, A16, A22, and B1–B5. Outbreaks of HFMD are usually caused by coxsackievirus A16.

Treatment

Self-limiting condition.

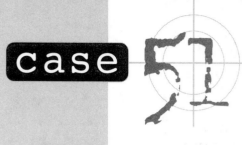

case 51

ID/CC	A 25-year-old homosexual man visits a health clinic complaining of headache, low-grade fever, and a **painful skin rash in the perianal area**.
HPI	He has no history of penile ulcerations and admits to **unprotected anal sex** with **multiple partners**.
PE	Perianal **vesicular** rash in clusters **on erythematous base**; no penile ulceration; painful inguinal lymphadenopathy.

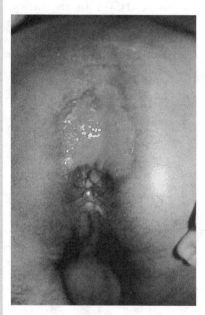

Figure 51-1. Severe erosive collesced perianal lesions.

Labs	**Multinucleated giant cells with intranuclear inclusions** surrounded by clear halo on Pap-stained section or Tzanck preparation of scrapings from base of vesicles.
Gross Pathology	Clear liquid in vesicles; secondary bacterial infection may result; painful ulcerations when vesicles rupture.
Micro Pathology	Inflammatory infiltrate with abundant lymphocytes.

VIROLOGY

case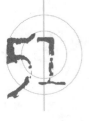

Herpes Genitalis

Differential | Chancroid
Chicken Pox
Syphilis
Drug Eruption
Herpes Zoster
Contact Dermatitis

Discussion | An enveloped, dsDNA virus transmitted by sexual contact, HSV-2 has a **tendency to recur** and can be **transmitted to the fetus through the birth canal.** Condom use appears to be one of the most effective means of preventing transmission.

Breakout Point |

> **Medically Important Double-stranded DNA Viruses:**
> - Papovavirus (unenveloped)
> - Adenovirus (unenveloped)
> - Hepadnovirus (enveloped)
> - Herpesvirus (enveloped)
> - Poxvirus (enveloped)

Treatment | **Acyclovir** for treating acute vesicular disease and reducing frequency of subsequent recurrent episodes.

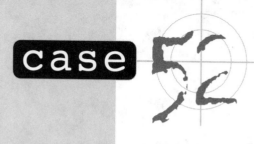
case 52

ID/CC A 30-year-old man presents with a **high fever** and chills, **headache, nausea,** vomiting, and muscle aches.

HPI Yesterday he had an episode involving abnormal movements of his right hand and face (FOCAL SEIZURE). He also has difficulty comprehending speech and has **olfactory hallucinations.** He has no history of psychiatric illness.

PE VS: fever; tachycardia; mild tachypnea; BP normal. PE: **confused and disoriented; papilledema;** mild nuchal rigidity; Kernig sign positive; paraphasic errors in speech; deep tendon reflexes normal and bilaterally symmetric.

Labs LP: cells 400/μL with **mononuclear pleocytosis;** mildly elevated protein; normal glucose; CSF PCR reveals **HSV type 1 (HSV-1);** serum complement-fixing antibody titer >1:1000. EEG: **spiked and slow waves localized to temporal lobes.**

Imaging MR: characteristic changes of **encephalitis** seen over medial **temporal lobes.**

Gross Pathology Hemorrhagic, necrotizing encephalitis most severe along inferior and medial regions of temporal lobes and orbitofrontal gyri.

Micro Pathology Brain biopsy reveals **Cowdry intranuclear viral inclusion bodies** in both neurons and glial cells with perivascular inflammatory infiltrates.

VIROLOGY

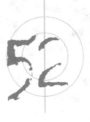

case

Herpes Simplex Encephalitis

Differential | Aseptic Meningitis
Complex Partial Seizure
Intracranial Abscess
Migraine Headache
Leptomeningeal Carcinomatosis
Intracranial Hemorrhage

Discussion | HSV can cause encephalitis. In the newborn, HSV-2 is usually the cause; after the neonatal period, most cases result from HSV-1. Neonatal infection (usually HSV-2) occurs after exposure to maternal genital infection at the time of delivery. The precise pathogenesis of HSV-1 encephalitis in the older child or the adult is not clear, but viral spread into the temporal lobe by both olfactory and trigeminal routes has been postulated.

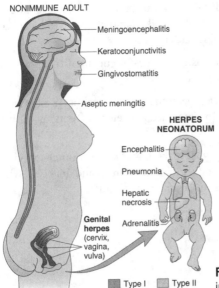

Figure 52-1. Herpes simplex infections.

Breakout Point

> HSV is the **most common cause of acute sporadic encephalitis** in the United States

Treatment | Intravenous acyclovir.

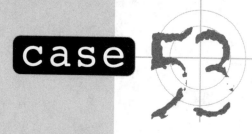

case 53

ID/CC A 45-year-old **HIV-positive** woman is seen by her family doctor following the appearance of a **painful, burning skin rash** on the **left side of her abdomen** that is accompanied by a headache and low-grade fever.

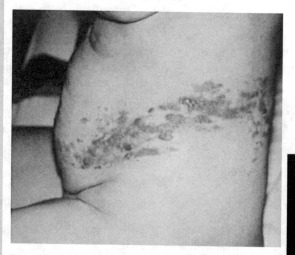

Figure 53-1. Painful, grouped vesicles in a unilateral dermatomal distribution.

HPI The patient had chickenpox as a child. She had been well until 1 year ago, when she was diagnosed with **non-Hodgkin lymphoma**, for which she is currently undergoing **chemotherapy**.

PE **Vesicular rash on erythematous base; in dermatomal distribution** (left T10–L1); exquisitely tender to touch.

Labs Acantholytic cells on **Tzanck smear** from base of **vesicles**.

Micro Pathology **Intranuclear eosinophilic inclusions surrounded by clear halo** (COWDRY A INCLUSIONS).

case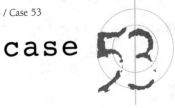

Herpes Zoster (Shingles)

Differential

Herpes Simplex
Impetigo
Smallpox
Atopic Dermatitis
Contact Dermatitis (Poison Ivy)

Discussion

Shingles represents a reactivation of a latent infection with **VZV**; the rash typically follows the distribution of a nerve root. It is commonly seen in **immunosuppressed patients** and is also associated with trauma, ultraviolet radiation, hypothermia, and **emotional stress**. Postherpetic neuralgia is a common complication in the elderly.

Breakout Point

> Patients with active shingles can infect naïve patients and cause chickenpox.

Treatment

Acyclovir.

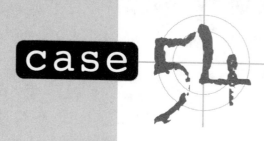
ID/CC   A 60-year-old man presents with **swelling and a vesicular skin eruption on the left side of his face.**

HPI   The patient reports that, before the rash developed, he had severe radiating pain on the left side of his face. He also recalls having suffered an attack of **chickenpox during his childhood.**

PE   **Unilateral vesicular rash** over left forehead and nasal bridge, including the tip of the nose, indicating involvement of the **nasociliary branch** of the trigeminal nerve (HUTCHINSON SIGN); skin of lids red and edematous; slit-lamp examination reveals numerous rounded spots composed of minute white dots involving epithelium and stroma, producing a **coarse subepithelial punctate keratitis; cornea** is **insensitive.**

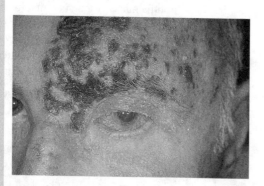

Figure 54-1. Crusting lesions on the forehead and scaling of the upper eyelid with conjunctival injection.

VIROLOGY

Micro Pathology   Vesicular skin lesions with **inclusions** that are **intranuclear and acidophilic** with a clear halo around them (**Cowdry type A inclusion bodies**); syncytial giant cells also seen.

107

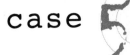 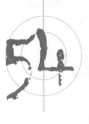

Herpes Zoster Ophthalmicus

Differential

Chemical Burn

Viral Conjunctivitis

Uveitic Glaucoma

Scleritis

HIV Ophthalmicus

Keratitis

Trigeminal Neuralgia

Discussion

Herpes zoster ophthalmicus is caused by the **VZV,** which causes chickenpox as a primary infection. Zoster is believed to be a **reactivation of the latent viral infection.** In **zoster ophthalmicus,** the chief **focus of reactivation is the trigeminal ganglion** from which the virus travels down one or more branches of the ophthalmic division such that its area of distribution is marked out by rows of vesicles or scars left by the vesicles. **Ocular complications** arise during subsidence of the rash and are generally **associated with** involvement of the **nasociliary branch** of the trigeminal nerve.

Treatment

Analgesic therapy; warm, moist compresses; early antiviral use (acyclovir, famciclovir, valacyclovir); antibiotics for secondary infection of vesicles.

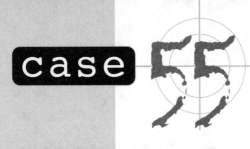

ID/CC An 8-month-old baby boy is brought to a pediatrician because of severe, intractable **chronic diarrhea** and **failure to thrive.**

HPI The **mother died of AIDS** shortly after the baby was delivered. The baby was **asymptomatic at birth.**

PE VS: fever; tachycardia. PE: emaciated, grossly malnourished; **oral thrush; generalized lymphadenopathy; hepatosplenomegaly.**

Labs **Decreased CD4 cell count;** increased serum immunoglobulin level with impaired production of specific antibodies.

VIROLOGY

109

case 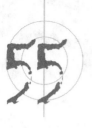 55

Human Immunodeficiency Virus Transmission in Pregnancy

Discussion

Vertical transmission of HIV-1 may occur in utero through **transplacental passage** of the virus, **during delivery,** or **postnatally through breast feeding**; however, it is believed that most infections are acquired at birth through contact with contaminated blood or secretions. Women who carry the virus should thus be discouraged from becoming pregnant or from breast feeding. The rate of transmission of HIV-1 from mother to infant has varied from 13% to 45%, with an average of 25%; however, when AZT is administered to HIV-1–infected pregnant women and to infants during the first 6 weeks of life, the risk of maternal-infant transmission is significantly reduced.

Breakout Point

HIV Testing in Neonates

ELISA and Western blot for HIV-1 positive (could be due to placental transfer of antibodies to HIV, but strongly supports diagnosis in presence of symptoms); PCR for **HIV RNA-positive** (confirming HIV infection).

Treatment

Nutritional support, *Pneumocystis carinii* prophylaxis, AZT (ZIDOVUDINE) therapy (suppresses replication by inhibiting viral reverse transcriptase), and anti-infective agents for specific infections; IV serum immunoglobulin to reduce frequency of bacterial infections; **oral polio vaccine and BCG contraindicated.**

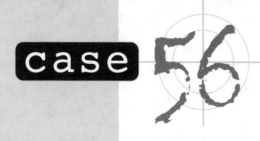

case 56

ID/CC An 18-year-old man complains of severe **irritation** in the left eye, **blurred vision**, excessive **lacrimation, and photophobia**.

HPI He reports that he has had **similar episodes** in the past that were treated with an antiviral drug. His records indicate that he suffered the **first attack** at the age of 7, at which time his condition was diagnosed and treated **as a severe follicular keratoconjunctivitis**; his records also indicate a history of recurrent episodes of **herpes labialis**.

PE Examination of left eye reveals circumcorneal congestion; fluorescein staining of cornea reveals infiltrates spreading in all directions, coalescing with each other and forming a **large, shallow ulcer with crenated edges** (DENDRITIC ULCER); **cornea** is **insensitive**.

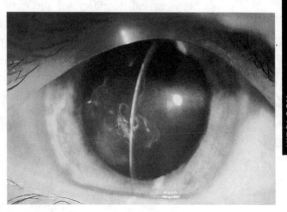

Figure 56-1. Patient with corneal scarring and reduced vision.

Labs **HSV-1** demonstrated on immunofluorescent staining of epithelial scrapings as well as in the aqueous humor.

VIROLOGY

case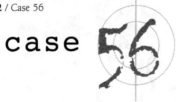

Herpes Simplex Virus Keratitis

Differential

Corneal Abrasion
Bacterial Keratitis
Fungal Keratitis
Corneal Ulcer
Keratoconjunctivitis Sicca

Discussion

Most ocular herpetic infections are **caused by HSV-1.** It is also the primary cause of corneal blindness in the United States. Primary infections present as unilateral follicular conjunctivitis, blepharitis, or corneal epithelial opacities; **recurrences** may take the **form of keratitis** (>90% of cases are unilateral), blepharitis, or keratoconjunctivitis. **Branching dendritic ulcers,** usually detected by fluorescein staining, are virtually diagnostic; deep stromal involvement may result in scarring, corneal thinning, and abnormal vascularization with resulting blindness or rupture of the globe.

Treatment

Analgesics; acyclovir; topical trifluridine or idoxuridine; antibiotics for secondary infections.

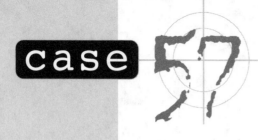
ID/CC A 38-year-old White woman visits her gynecologist for a **routine Pap smear.**

HPI She admits to early sexual activity, **many sexual partners,** and **unprotected sex.**

PE Pallor; cervical tenderness; a few small, raised, flat lesions on cervix; **genital warts** also seen on vulva (CONDYLOMATA ACUMINATA).

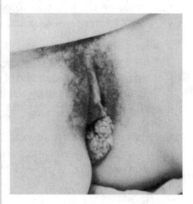

Figure 57-1. Large vulvar and perianal genital warts.

Labs Presence of HPV in cervical cells revealed on **DNA hybridization and immunofluorescent antibody assays** for viral antigen.

Micro Pathology Rounded basophilic cells on Pap smear with **large nuclei** occupying most of surface; **nuclei show mitoses and coarse clumping of chromatin with perinuclear halo** (SEVERE KOILOCYTIC DYSPLASIA).

VIROLOGY

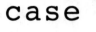 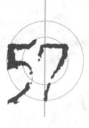

Human Papillomavirus

Differential

Cervical Cancer

Hidradenitis

Malignant Vulvar Lesion

Molluscum Contagiosum

Discussion

Infection with **HPV types 16, 18, and 31** is strongly associated with **cervical cancer** preceded by dysplasia. Spread of the infection to partners may be prevented by barrier contraception.

Breakout Point

> HPV viral protein E6 interferes with cellular p53 and E7 leads to dysfunction of cellular retinoblastoma (Rb), leading to cellular transformation.

Treatment

Cryotherapy, conization, or local excision with follow-up. A vaccine has recently been introduced for women, 9 to 26 years of age. It protects against HPV **Types 6, 11, 16, and 18.**

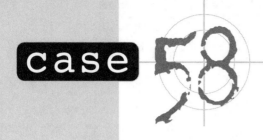

case 58

ID/CC	A 57-year-old **Black** man complains to his doctor of increasing weakness, **swollen glands in the armpits and groin,** and a feeling of **heaviness in the abdomen** (due to hepatosplenomegaly).
HPI	The patient is an immigrant from **Trinidad and Tobago** and has a history of nonresolving skin rashes and recurrent respiratory infections.
PE	Marked **pallor;** extensive papular skin rash with few erythematous plaques over abdomen; **generalized lymphadenopathy and hepatosplenomegaly.**
Labs	CBC/PBS: marked **leukocytosis** (83000) with relative **lymphocytosis** and **atypical lymphocytes. Increased LDH; hypercalcemia;** ELISA negative for HIV.
Imaging	CXR: normal.
Micro Pathology	Skin biopsy reveals infiltration by **leukemic CD4 T lymphocytes** with the formation of **Pautrier microabscess.**

VIROLOGY

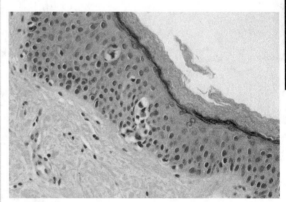

Figure 58-1. Pautrier microabscess.

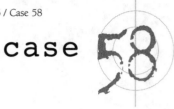

case

Human T-Cell Leukemia Virus Type 1

Differential

Human Immunodeficiency Syndrome

Non-Hodgkin Lymphoma

Syphilis

Discussion

ATLL is associated with HTLV-1 type C, a retrovirus that has a higher incidence in **Blacks** from the **Caribbean and southeastern United States** as well as in people from **southern Japan and sub-Saharan Africa**. The infection is acquired via transmission from mother to child (breast milk), from sexual activity, from blood transfusion, or from IV drug use.

Treatment

Aggressive combination chemotherapy.

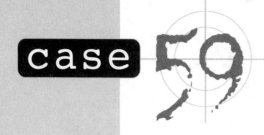

ID/CC A 20-year-old man studying in college complains of **sore throat, fatigue, fever, swollen lymph nodes on the back of his neck,** anorexia, cough, and **malaise** of 10 days' duration.

HPI He was initially given **ampicillin** by his school nurse, after which he developed an extensive **skin rash.**

PE VS: fever. PE: enlargement of submaxillary and **cervical lymph nodes; exudative tonsillitis;** petechiae on soft palate; slightly **enlarged spleen and liver.**

Labs CBC/PBS: anemia; thrombocytopenia; leukocytosis with absolute **lymphocytosis** (50%); **atypical lymphocytes.** Elevated ALT, AST, and bilirubin; **positive heterophil antibody test** (MONOSPOT TEST); IgM antibodies to viral capsid antigen positive.

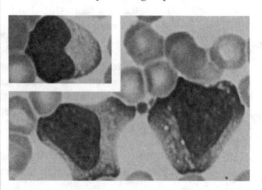

Figure 59-1. Atypical lymphocytes.

Gross Pathology Enlarged spleen, lymph nodes, and, to lesser extent, liver; hepatitis may be present along with brain involvement; splenic rupture rare complication.

Micro Pathology Proliferation of reticuloendothelial system; infiltration of spleen by atypical lymphocytes.

VIROLOGY

117

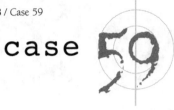

case

Infectious Mononucleosis

Differential

Human Immunodeficiency Syndrome
Mumps
Rubella
Scarlet Fever
Pharyngitis
CMV Infection

Discussion

Infectious mononucleosis is a systemic viral infection that is caused by EBV, a herpesvirus, and is transmitted through respiratory droplets and saliva. In developed countries, it most commonly affects teenagers and young adults ("kissing disease"); in underdeveloped countries, it is seen as a subclinical infection of early childhood. EBV infection is associated with an increased risk of **Burkitt lymphoma**, **Hodgkin disease**, and **nasopharyngeal carcinoma**.

Breakout Point

> **Heterophil antibodies** are antibodies to sheep RBCs. Patients with EBV infectious mononucleosis make heterophil antibodies, whereas those with CMV infectious mononucleosis do not.

Treatment

Supportive; avoid contact sports until resolution of splenomegaly to protect against rupture.

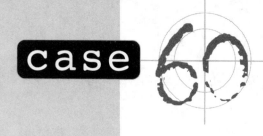
case 60

ID/CC   A 65-year-old man presents with a **high fever**, head-ache, extreme prostration, a **nonproductive cough**, and severe **breathlessness**.

HPI   He had been receiving chlorambucil for treatment of CLL and was in an extremely **debilitated state**.

PE   VS: fever; tachypnea; cyanosis. PE: **conjunctival congestion; pharyngeal inflammation; rales and wheezes** heard on auscultation over both lung fields; splenomegaly and lymphadenopathy (due to CLL).

Labs   No organisms seen or cultured from sputum; fluorescent antibody directed against **influenza virus** was positive; viral cultures of nasopharyngeal washings grew influenza virus; fourfold rise in **hemagglutination inhibition antibody titer** against influenza virus demonstrated.

Imaging CXR (PA view): bilateral, diffuse interstitial infiltrates suggestive of **atypical pneumonia**.

case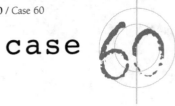

Influenza

Differential

Adenovirus Infection

Infectious Mononucleosis

Parainfluenza Infection

Rhinovirus Infection

Atypical Pneumonia

Discussion

Influenza viruses are medium-sized spherical **RNA viruses termed orthomyxoviruses**; influenza A and B viruses each contain 8 RNA segments and 10 viral proteins. Influenza infection is **most common in winter**, with the **severity** of a given **outbreak depending on the status of immunity** in the community. Previous natural infection or immunization with viruses that are immunologically close to the current strain limits new infection, but if **antigenic drift** results in reduced cross-reactivity, the new strain will spread more rapidly. New strains produced by **antigenic shift** account for most major outbreaks. Influenza affects all segments of the population, but severe infections and **major complications** are most common **in patients who are young, elderly, or debilitated.**

Treatment

Amantadine or rimantadine for influenza A (**zanamivir or oseltamivir** for influenza A and B); ventilatory support, antipyretics, and IV fluids. **Secondary staphylococcal pneumonia** should be treated with parenteral antibiotics; **yearly vaccination** prevents excessive morbidity and mortality, especially among the elderly.

Breakout Point

> The influenza vaccines, both live and attenuated, contain a preparation of **23 subtypes** and are formulated each year based on projected epidemiologic data on the prevalent strains.

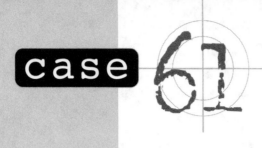

case 67

ID/CC A 30-year-old man, a **laboratory researcher** presents with a **high fever, neck rigidity**, retro-orbital pain, and severe myalgias of a few days' duration.

HPI The patient also complains of a **sore throat** and photophobia. His work in the lab involves **close contact with** experimental animals such as **hamsters, white mice, and nude mice.** He was adequately vaccinated.

PE VS: fever. PE: neck stiffness and **Kernig sign positive** (due to meningeal irritation); pharyngeal inflammation but no exudate noted.

Labs CBC: mild leukopenia. LP: CSF suggestive of **aseptic meningitis.**

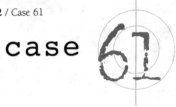

case 61

Lymphocytic Choriomeningitis

Differential

Enterovirus Infection

Amebic Meningoencephalitis

Herpes Virus Encephalitis

West Nile Virus encephalitis

Bacterial Meningitis

Discussion

LCM virus is an **arenavirus.** Sporadic cases occur after **infection from feral mice,** but the **most common sources** of human infection are **pet/lab rodents.** The virus is considered a **major lab hazard,** and care must be taken to avoid accidental infection. There is **no** commercially available **vaccine.**

Breakout Point

Single-stranded (-) RNA Viruses

- Orthomyxovirus
- Paramyxovirus
- Rhabdovirus
- Filovirus
- Arenavirus
- Bunyavirus

Treatment

Supportive; ribavirin may play a role.

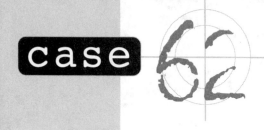

ID/CC A **3-year-old** boy is brought to the ER with a **high fever of 7 days' duration,** accompanied by **redness of the eyes,** persistent dry **cough,** and **coryza.**

HPI His family doctor had treated his illness as a viral URI, but no improvement was seen. One day before his admission, his mother noticed a **skin rash starting behind his ears and face** that has now spread to his trunk and extremities.

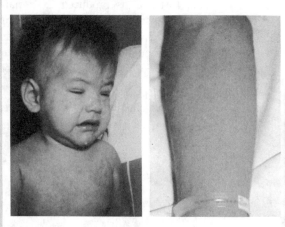

Figure 62-1. Patient on presentation.

PE Pallor; injected conjunctiva; hyperemic throat; erythematous maculopapular rash on face, neck, trunk, and extremities; retroauricular lymphadenopathy; **bluish-gray spots surrounded by erythematous areola on buccal mucosa in region of first molar** (KOPLIK SPOTS).

Labs CBC: **leukopenia.**

Micro Pathology Lymphocytic dermal infiltration; multinucleated giant cells in reticuloendothelial system (WARTHIN-FINKELDEY CELLS).

case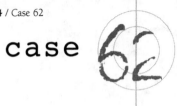

Measles

Differential

Enterovirus Infection

Kawasaki Disease

Parvovirus B19 Infection

Rubella

Scalded Skin Syndrome

Discussion

Also called **rubeola**; not to be confused with rubella. Measles is produced by a **paramyxovirus** and is transmitted by **respiratory droplets**; a live attenuated vaccine is available. Measles has an incubation period of 10 to 14 days. Sequelae include encephalitis, SSPE, and giant cell pneumonia.

Treatment

No specific antiviral therapy available; vitamin A supplementation may be helpful; treat complications.

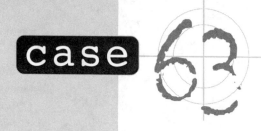
ID/CC　A 30-year-old homosexual man visits his family doctor complaining of a nonpruritic **skin eruption** on his **upper limbs, trunk,** and **anogenital area.**

HPI　He has been **HIV positive** for about 3 years and admits to having continued unprotected intercourse.

PE　Multiple painless, pearly-white, dome-shaped, waxy, **umbilicated nodules** 2 to 5 mm in diameter on arms, trunk, and anogenital area; **palms and soles spared.**

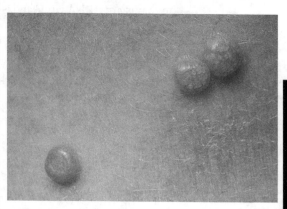

Figure 63-1. Flesh-colored nodules with a mosaic surface and central umbilication.

Gross Pathology　Firm, umbilicated nodules containing thick yellowish material.

Micro Pathology　Stained histologic sections confirm diagnosis with large **cytoplasmic inclusions** in material expressed from lesions.

VIROLOGY

125

case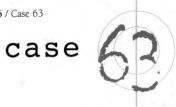

Molluscum Contagiosum

Differential
Basal Cell Carcinoma
Condyloma Acuminatum
Chicken Pox
Atopic Dermatitis
Herpes Simplex

Discussion
Molluscum contagiosum is a benign, autoinoculable skin disease of children and young adults; it is caused by a poxvirus (DNA virus) and is transmitted through sexual contact, close bodily contact, clothing, or towels. It is one of many opportunistic infections seen in patients with AIDS (difficult to eradicate).

Treatment
Lesions may resolve spontaneously or be removed by curettage, cryotherapy, or podophyllin; no antiviral drug or vaccine available.

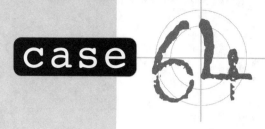
ID/CC A **6-year-old** White man presents with fever, nausea, vomiting, **swelling**, and tenderness of the **mandibular angle**; he finds it difficult to talk, eat, or swallow.

HPI Two of his classmates were diagnosed with mumps 2 weeks ago. There is no vaccination record available.

PE VS: fever. PE: outward and upward displacement of ear; **obliterated mandibular hollow; orifice of Stensen duct swollen and hyperemic; right testicle enlarged and painful.**

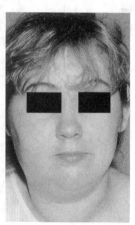

Figure 64-1. Bilateral parotitis.

VIROLOGY

Labs CBC: leukopenia with **lymphocytosis. Hyperamylasemia;** positive complement fixation antibodies.

Gross Pathology Parotid glands enlarged with areas of necrosis and mononuclear infiltrate; encephalitis, orchitis, oophoritis, meningitis, and pancreatitis may also be present.

Micro Pathology Examination of parotid glands reveals perivascular mononuclear, lymphocytic, and plasma cell infiltrate with necrosis; ductal obstruction and edema; testicular interstitial edema; perivascular cerebral lymphocytic cuffing.

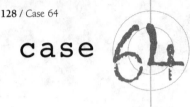

case

Mumps

Differential
Viral Parotitis
Bacterial Parotitis
Calculus of the Stensen Duct
Salivary Gland Tumor
Mikulicz Syndrome

Discussion
A systemic infection caused by the mumps virus, an RNA paramyxovirus, mumps is transmitted by droplets and direct contact. Bilateral testicular involvement may lead to sterility; one of the most common causes of pancreatitis in children. A vaccine is available with measles and rubella (MMR).

Treatment
Supportive; analgesics for pain; treat complications.

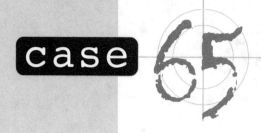

case 65

ID/CC	A **25-year-old man** complains of increasing **shortness of breath** and **ankle edema** that have progressively worsened over the past 2 weeks.
HPI	He also complains of fatigue, palpitations, and low-grade fever. His symptoms **followed a severe URI**. He denies any history of joint pain or skin rash (vs. rheumatic fever).
PE	JVP elevated; pitting pedal edema; fine inspiratory crepitations heard at both lung bases; mild hepatosplenomegaly.
Labs	ASO titers not elevated. CBC: lymphocytosis. ECG: first-degree AV block. ESR elevated; increased titers of antibodies to **coxsackievirus** demonstrated in serum.
Imaging	CXR: **cardiomegaly** and **pulmonary edema.** Echo: **dilated cardiomyopathy with low ejection fraction.**
Gross Pathology	Dilated heart with foci of epicardial, myocardial, and endocardial petechial hemorrhages.
Micro Pathology	Endomyocardial biopsy reveals **diffuse infiltration by mononuclear cells,** predominantly lymphocytes; focal fibrosis.

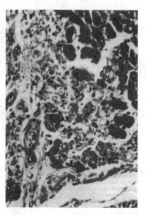

Figure 65-1. Myocardial biopsy showing extensive inflammatory cellular infiltrate with myocyte necrosis.

case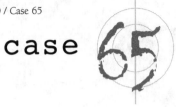

Viral Myocarditis

Differential

Amyloidosis

Cardiac Tumor

Endocardial Fibroelastosis

Rheumatic Heart Disease

Dressler Syndrome

Discussion

Coxsackie B is most often implicated in viral myocarditis. Nonviral causes of myocarditis include bacteria such as *Borrelia burgdorferi* (Lyme disease), parasites such as *Trypanosoma cruzi* (Chagas disease), hypersensitivity reaction (SLE, drug reaction), radiation, and sarcoidosis; may also be idiopathic (giant cell myocarditis).

Treatment

Manage CHF and arrhythmias; cardiac transplant in intractable cases.

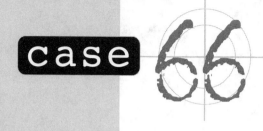

case 66

ID/CC A 15-year-old man presents with **painful bilateral swelling of the parotid glands,** left-sided scrotal pain, and fever.

HPI Nothing in the patient's history suggests that he had childhood mumps. He has not received all his vaccinations.

PE VS: fever. PE: bilateral parotid gland enlargement with obliteration of mandibular hollow; hyperemia and edema of Stensen duct (parotid duct) orifice; retroauricular lymphadenopathy; left-sided scrotal and **testicular swelling with tenderness.**

Labs CBC: leukopenia with **lymphocytosis; hyperamylasemia.**

Imaging US, scrotum: increased color flow and edema.

Gross Pathology Enlarged, edematous testicle.

Micro Pathology Parotid glands show perivascular mononuclear, lymphocytic, and plasma cell infiltrate with necrosis; ductal obstruction and edema; testicular interstitial edema; perivascular cerebral lymphocytic cuffing.

case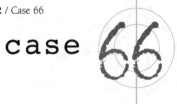

Orchitis

Differential

Epididymitis

Hernia (direct or indirect)

Testicular Torsion

Hydrocele

Testicular Tumor

Discussion

Orchitis may be caused by bacterial infections such as *Escherichia coli* and other enterobacteria; viral infections such as **mumps**; STDs such as *Chlamydia* species or gonorrhea; or pathogens such as *Mycobacterium tuberculosis*. Mumps orchitis may give rise to sterility if bilateral.

■ TABLE 66-1 COMPARISON OF EPIDIDYMITIS, ORCHITIS, AND TORSION OF THE TESTICLE

Factor	Epididymitis	Orchitis	Torsion
Age	Adolescent	Postpubertal	Prepubertal/ adolescent
Common cause	Viral, chemicals, STD	Viral (mumps)	Bell clapper deformity
Bilaterality	Unusual	20%–60%	Almost never
Dysuria	Often +	Usually −	Usually −
Fever	+ / −	+	Usually −
Nausea/vomiting	+ / −	+ / −	+ / −
Onset	Gradual	1−2 days	Sudden
Localized pain	Epididymis (early)	Entire testicle	Testis, abdomen, flank
Urinalysis	+/− WBCs	+/− WBCs	Usually no WBCs
Cremaster reflex	Usually present	Usually present	Usually absent
Doppler	Increased flow	Increased flow	Decreased flow

Treatment

Scrotal support; analgesics, ice packs; corticosteroids.

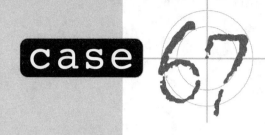
case 67

ID/CC   A 35-year-old man complains of **fever, nonproductive cough,** and **chest pain.**

HPI   He states that the chest pain developed after he had a severe cold for 1 week. He describes the pain as **severe, crushing, and constant** over the anterior chest and adds that it **worsens with inspiration** and is **relieved by sitting up** and bending forward.

PE   VS: low-grade fever; sinus tachycardia. PE: triphasic **pericardial friction rub** (systolic and diastolic components followed by a third component in late diastole associated with atrial contraction); **elevated JVP;** inappropriate **increase in JVP with inspiration** (KUSSMAUL SIGN); pulsus paradoxus may also be seen.

Labs   Moderately elevated transaminases and LDH; **elevated ESR; serum CPK-MB normal.** CBC: neutrophilic leukocytosis. ECG: **diffuse ST-segment elevation** (vs. MI); **PR-segment depression.**

Imaging   Echo: **pericardial effusion.** CXR: apparent **cardiomegaly** (due to effusion).

Gross Pathology   In long-standing cases, pericardium may become fibrotic, scarred, and calcified.

Micro Pathology   Pericardial biopsy reveals signs of acute inflammation with increased leukocytes, vascularity, and deposition of fibrin.

VIROLOGY

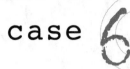

case

Pericarditis

Differential

Aortic Dissection
Esophageal Rupture
Esophagitis
Gastritis
MI

Discussion

Acute pericarditis is commonly idiopathic. Known infectious causes include **coxsackievirus A and B, tuberculosis,** staphylococcal or pneumococcal infection, amebiasis, or actinomycosis; noninfectious causes include chronic renal failure, **collagen vascular disease** (SLE, scleroderma, and rheumatoid arthritis), neoplasms, MI, and trauma. Long-term sequelae include chronic constrictive pericarditis.

Breakout Point

> **Causes of Pericarditis are CARDIAC RIND**
>
> **C**ollagen vascular disease
> **A**ortic aneurysm
> **R**adiation
> **D**rugs
> **I**nfections
> **A**cute renal failure
> **C**ardiac infarction
> **R**heumatic fever
> **I**njury
> **N**eoplasms
> **D**ressler syndrome

Treatment

Analgesics for pain; steroids in resistant cases; indomethacin; surgical stripping of scarring in severe cases.

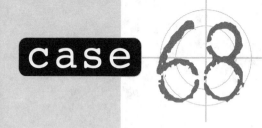

ID/CC A 3-year-old man, the child of recent African immigrants, is brought to the local health center because of **asymmetrical legs**.

HPI His parents give a history of **incomplete immunization**. They add that 5 months ago the boy had **fever and diarrhea** that subsided spontaneously; a few weeks later they noted that he could not use his right leg.

PE Right leg **thin, short, wasted, weak, and flaccid; absent deep tendon reflexes** in right leg; **no sensory deficit**; upper limbs normal; mental status and CNs normal.

Labs EMG: chronic partial denervation with abnormal spontaneous activity in resting muscle and reduction in number of motor units under voluntary control; normal sensory conduction studies.

Micro Pathology Widespread inflammation, mainly in the anterior horn.

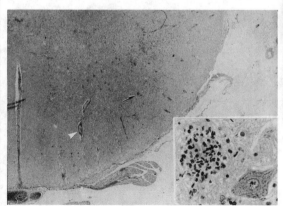

Figure 68-1. Perivascular cuff of chronic inflammatory cells (*white arrowhead*) and neuronophagia (*black arrow*) are apparent.

VIROLOGY

case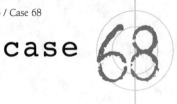

Poliomyelitis

Differential

Botulism

Tetanus

Rabies

Aseptic Meningitis

Guillain-Barré Syndrome

Discussion

A symptomatic disease caused by poliovirus that is more common in infants and children, poliomyelitis can result in muscular atrophy and skeletal deformity. It attacks motor neurons in the anterior horns and may affect CNs (bulbar polio); it is preventable by vaccine.

Treatment

Rehabilitation, supportive.

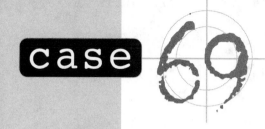
ID/CC A 26-year-old nurse presented with headaches and **recent-onset seizures;** she also complained of increasing **right-sided numbness and blurring of vision.**

HPI A clinical diagnosis of HSV encephalitis had previously been made, for which the patient was treated with 2 courses of acyclovir without any amelioration of symptoms; the **disease continued to progress** both radiologically and clinically. On serology she tested **HIV positive.**

PE Neurologic exam reveals **cognitive mental impairment; visual field defects and sensory dysphasia** seen; **an ill-defined sensory loss** on right side of body.

Labs HIV positive by ELISA and Western blot.

Imaging MR (T2-weighted): patchy high-intensity lesions **in the deep white matter of both cerebral hemispheres** involving temporal, parietal, and occipital lobes.

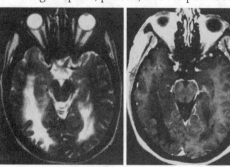

Figure 69-1. MR image shows increased signal intensity of the temporooccipital white matter with relative cortical sparing.

Micro Pathology Stereotactic biopsy sections show abnormal brain with rarefaction, numerous reactive astrocytes, foamy histiocytes, and inflammatory infiltrate around some vessels; **JC virus in situ hybridization** shows many **positive nuclei;** no herpesvirus inclusions seen; **electron microscopy** demonstrates cells with **typical papovavirus** structures in nucleus.

VIROLOGY

137

case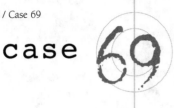

Progressive Multifocal Leukoencephalopathy

Differential | Toxoplasmosis
HIV Encephalitis
Multiple Sclerosis
CNS Lymphoma
Postradiation Change

Discussion | PML is a **progressive demyelinating disease related to JC papovavirus infection;** the largest number of cases occur in **persons who are immunocompromised** for any of a variety of reasons, including organ transplantation, hematologic and other malignant diseases, chronic immunosuppressive therapy, and AIDS.

Treatment | Disease was **relentlessly progressive** and resulted in **death within 6 months.**

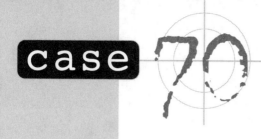

ID/CC A 12-year-old White woman is rushed to the ER because of **numbness** of the right foot and leg followed by **fever** and **convulsions**. The child **refuses to drink any fluids** (HYDROPHOBIA).

HPI She had been camping 5 weeks ago. When questioned, her mother recalls that one night the child had apparently stepped on **a bat that bit her in the right foot**.

PE VS: no fever. PE: child is **disoriented, hyperventilating,** extremely agitated, and actively moving all four limbs, thus **difficult to restrain;** no meningeal signs; fundus normal; **saliva viscous and foaming**.

Labs LP: lymphocytic pleocytosis with mildly elevated proteins and normal sugar in CSF; RFFIT positive for rabies antibodies.

Micro Pathology Characteristic **cytoplasmic inclusion bodies** (NEGRI BODIES) in **nuchal skin biopsy, corneal scrapings,** and **Ammon horn**.

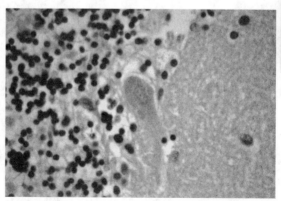

Figure 70-1. Intracytoplasmic inclusions (Negri bodies).

VIROLOGY

case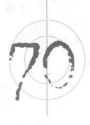

Rabies

Differential

Poliomyelitis

Tetanus

Transverse Myelitis

Psychosis

Guillain-Barré Syndrome

Creutzfeldt-Jakob Disease

Atropine Poisoning

Discussion

Rabies is a fatal viral disease that is transmitted to humans by the bites of **bats, raccoons,** skunks, foxes, coyotes, dogs, and cats. Rabies virus is an enveloped, single-stranded RNA virus. Rabies has a **long incubation period** (approximately 3 to 8 weeks); death usually results from respiratory failure.

Treatment

Supportive; almost always fatal; prevent with vaccine; postexposure prophylaxis with diploid cell vaccine and HRIG.

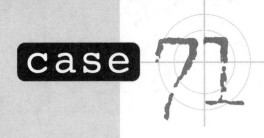
ID/CC   A 68-year-old man is seen with complaints of a **rash** along with **pain in his left ear** and inability to move the muscles of his face with accompanying asymmetry.

HPI   He suffered an attack of **chickenpox during childhood** but has no history either of a similar rash over his face or of any visual sign.

PE   **Vesicular rash** over left pinna (OTITIS EXTERNA); left-sided lower motor neuron-type **facial nerve palsy** (patient is unable to frown and unable to blink left eye; eyeballs roll up during attempt to close eye; patient is unable to whistle; taste sensation over anterior two-thirds of tongue lost on left side).

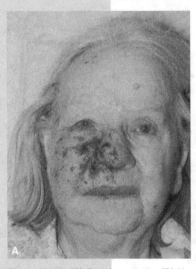
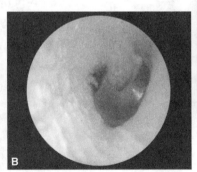

Figure 71-1. (A) Facial paralysis. **(B)** Herpetic vesicle on the tympanic membrane.

Gross Pathology   Neuritis and vesicular skin lesions confined to distribution of geniculate ganglion of facial nerve.

Micro Pathology   Vesicular skin lesions with **herpes viral inclusions,** i.e., intranuclear, acidophil inclusions with a halo around them (COWDRY TYPE A INCLUSIONS); syncytial cells also seen.

VIROLOGY

case 71

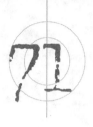

Ramsay-Hunt Syndrome

Differential

Bell Palsy

Postherpetic Neuralgia

Trigeminal Neuralgia

Temporomandibular Joint Syndrome

Discussion

Herpes zoster of the **geniculate ganglion,** or Ramsay-Hunt syndrome, presents as a vesicular rash on the pinna followed by ipsilateral LMN facial nerve palsy.

Breakout Point

Herpes Virus Family Members

- HSV-1
- HSV-2
- VZV
- CMV
- EBV
- HSV-6 **(sixth disease)**
- HSV-8 **(KSHV)**

Treatment

Systemic steroids and **acyclovir** are mainstays of management.

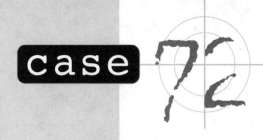
ID/CC An **18-month-old** boy is brought to the pediatrician following the appearance of an extensive skin rash.

HPI Four days ago he suddenly developed a **very high fever** (40°C) with no other symptoms or signs. The fever continued for 4 days until the day of his admission, when it abruptly **disappeared, coinciding with the onset of the rash.**

PE **Child looks well;** in no acute distress; **generalized rash** apparent as discrete 2-mm to 5-mm **rose-pink macules and papules on trunk, neck, and extremities** (face is spared); lesions blanch on pressure; no lymphadenopathy; splenomegaly may also be present.

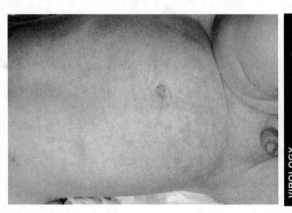

Figure 72-1. Characteristic rash.

Labs CBC/PBS: WBCs variable; relative lymphocytosis with atypical lymphocytes.

case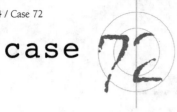

Roseola Infantum

Differential

Measles

Rubella

Erythema Infectiosum

Drug Eruption

Sepsis

Meningococcemia

Discussion

Roseola infantum, also called **exanthem subitum,** is caused by **human herpesvirus 6 (HHV-6).** It is the most common exanthematous disease in infants 2 years of age or younger and is a frequent cause of **febrile convulsions.**

Breakout Point

> Fifth disease (erythema infectiosum) is due to parvovirus B19.
> Sixth disease **(roseola infantum) is due to HHV-6.**

Treatment

Supportive; foscarnet in a few selected cases.

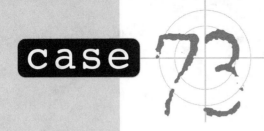
ID/CC A **10-month-old** boy presents with fever and severe **vomiting** followed by **watery diarrhea.**

HPI His stools are loose and watery without blood or mucus.

PE VS: fever; tachycardia. PE: child is irritable; moderate dehydration.

Labs Absence of leukocytes on fecal stain; rotavirus detected with **ELISA; electron microscopy** with negative staining identifies **viral particles** on stool ultrafiltrates.

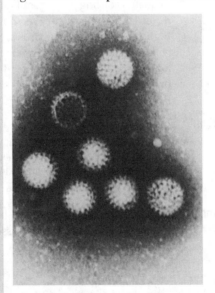

Figure 73-1. Particles observed by negative-stain electron microscopy in a stool suspension of a child with diarrhea.

Micro Pathology Major histopathologic lesions are characterized by reversible involvement of the proximal small intestine; mucosa remains intact with shortening of villi, a mixed inflammatory infiltration of lamina propria, and hyperplasia of the mucosal crypt cells; electron microscopy reveals distended cisterns of endoplasmic reticulum, mitochondrial swelling, and sparse, irregular microvilli.

VIROLOGY

case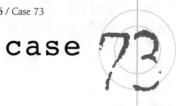

Rotavirus Diarrhea

Differential

Dehydration

Bacterial Gastroenteritis

Cholera

Salmonella

Discussion

Rotavirus group A is the single **most important cause** of endemic, **severe diarrheal illness in infants and young children worldwide**; it occurs with greater frequency during winter months in temperate climates and during the dry season in tropical climates. In the United States, rotavirus accounts for 50% of all childhood diarrheas, has an incubation period of 48 hours, is transmitted by the fecal-oral route, and lasts only a few days. Some children subsequently develop lactose intolerance, which lasts for a few weeks.

Breakout Point

Diarrheal diseases are a leading cause of child mortality; it is estimated that 600000 children worldwide die of rotaviral diarrhea.

Treatment

Fluid replacement therapy. A live, oral pentavalent vaccine that contains 5 live reassortant rotaviruses is now available.

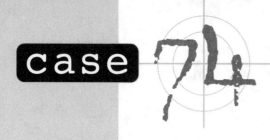

case 74

<table>
<tr><td>ID/CC</td><td>A 5-month-old baby boy is brought to the pediatric clinic with wheezing and respiratory difficulty of 3 hours' duration.</td></tr>
<tr><td>HPI</td><td>He has had rhinorrhea, fever, and cough and had been sneezing for 2 days prior to his visit to the clinic.</td></tr>
<tr><td>PE</td><td>VS: tachypnea. PE: nasal flaring; mild central cyanosis; accessory muscle use during respiration; hyperexpansion of chest; expiratory and inspiratory wheezes; rhonchi over both lung fields.</td></tr>
<tr><td>Labs</td><td>CBC/PBS: relative lymphocytosis. ABGs: hypoxemia with mild hypercapnia. Normal flora on bacterial culture of sputum.</td></tr>
<tr><td>Imaging</td><td>CXR: hyperinflation; segmental atelectasis; interstitial infiltrates.</td></tr>
<tr><td>Micro Pathology</td><td>Formation of giant multinucleated cells.</td></tr>
</table>

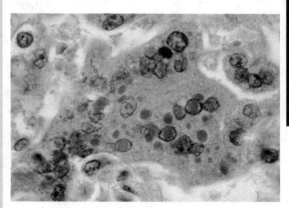

Figure 74-1. Giant cell (syncytia).

VIROLOGY

147

case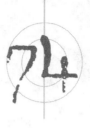

Respiratory Syncytial Virus Pneumonia

Differential

Asthma
Bronchiolitis
Croup
Influenza
Pneumonia

Discussion

RSV is the **most common cause of bronchiolitis in infants** under 2 years of age; other viral causes include parainfluenza, influenza, and adenovirus. Infections typically occur during the fall and winter months. Transmission occurs via close contact with contaminated fomites but can also occur after coughing or sneezing. The majority of infections occur during an RSV epidemic.

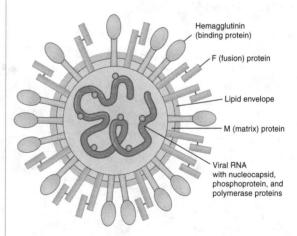

Figure 74-2. Schematic diagram of a paramyxovirus.

Treatment

Humidified oxygen; bronchodilators; aerosolized **ribavirin** for patients with severe infection.

ID/CC   A 10-year-old Asian immigrant woman presents with a **low-grade fever** and coryza of 3 days' duration.

HPI   She also complains of arthralgias and a **skin rash that began on her face and spread to her trunk.** Her mother says she cannot remember any details of her vaccination history.

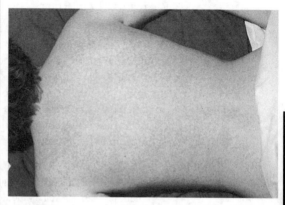

Figure 75-1. Top-to-bottom spread of discrete pink macules on the trunk.

PE   VS: fever. PE: maculopapular rash over face and trunk; **enlarged postauricular, posterior cervical, and occipital lymph nodes.**

Labs   CBC: leukopenia; thrombocytopenia.

Gross Pathology   Erythematous skin rash resembling rubeola measles but lighter in color and more discrete; similar distribution pattern in both.

case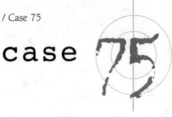

Rubella (German Measles)

Differential

Contact Dermatitis

Herpes Virus 6 Infection

Measles

Mononucleosis

Mycoplasma Infection

Parvovirus B19 Infection

Discussion

Rubella (German measles) is caused by a togavirus. Live attenuated rubella virus vaccine (part of MMR) should be given to all infants and to susceptible girls before menarche. The course of illness is self-limiting and mild; in females the major implication is the potential for congenital rubella syndrome. Females with rubella can get **polyarthritis** secondary to immune complex deposition.

Breakout Point

> The MMR vaccine is contraindicated for pregnant females as well as those who are immunosuppressed.

Treatment

Symptomatic treatment.

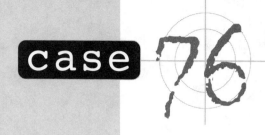

ID/CC A 4-month-old girl brought in for a well-child visit is found to be **low in weight and height for her age** and to have **lens opacities** (due to congenital cataracts).

HPI Her mother had a skin rash and fever during her **first trimester of pregnancy.** The mother states that when the child was born, she too had a **rash** like a "blueberry muffin" and was **jaundiced.**

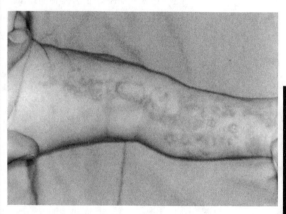

Figure 76-1. Diffuse, purplish papules and nodules create a blueberry-muffin appearance in an infant.

PE **Deaf** and **globally retarded**; malnourished; **microcephaly** and bulging anterior fontanelle; **microphthalmia** with unilateral left **cataract**; discrete black, patchy pigmentation found in retina on funduscopic exam; **hepatosplenomegaly**; **machinery murmur heard at second intercostal space** on left sternal border (due to **PDA**).

Labs CBC/PBS: leukopenia; thrombocytopenia. Increased serum bilirubin (both direct and indirect)

Imaging XR, plain: radiolucent (lytic) bone lesions (metaphyseal). Echo: PDA.

VIROLOGY

case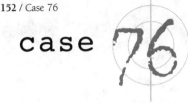

Rubella—Congenital

Differential
DiGeorge Syndrome
Neuroblastoma
Congenital Toxoplasmosis
Trisomy
Teratogen Exposure

Discussion
Congenital rubella, transmitted in utero, is caused by rubella virus, a single-stranded RNA togavirus. In children and adults it is a transitory and unremarkable disease. If acquired **in utero, it has devastating consequences.**

Treatment
Supportive; surgery for correction of congenital heart disease, cataracts, and glaucoma.

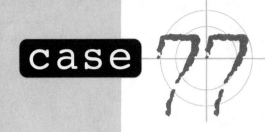
ID/CC   The case of a **12-year-old boy** who **died of a progressive degenerative neurologic disease** was discussed at an autopsy meeting.

HPI   The child had been developing normally up to 10 years of age, when his teachers noted a **progressive deterioration in intellect and personality;** this was followed by the development of **seizures akin to myoclonus,** signs of pyramidal and extrapyramidal disease, and finally a **state of decerebrate rigidity.** The child **died 7 months after the onset** of symptoms. His history revealed that he had had a **severe attack of measles at the age of 2.**

Labs   LP: routine CSF profile normal. **Gamma globulin level elevated;** markedly **elevated levels of measles antibody** present in both serum and CSF; despite the elevated antibody titers, **antibody to the M protein was not present.** EEG: pattern of **burst suppression and biphasic sharp and slow waves.**

Imaging   MR: nonspecific parenchymal abnormalities.

Micro Pathology   Histopathologically, the encephalitis involved both white and gray matter and was marked by lymphocytic infiltration, nerve cell degeneration, and demyelination; measles antigen demonstrated by immunofluorescence analysis, and particles resembling paramyxovirus were detected by electron microscopy.

VIROLOGY

case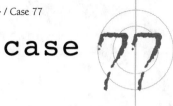

Subacute Sclerosing Panencephalitis (SSPE)

Differential

Brain Abscess
Leptospirosis
Toxoplasmosis
Meningitis
Tuberculosis.

Discussion

SSPE is caused by a **defective** (major defect is the lack or altered expression of the M-matrix protein) form of **measles virus** (family Paramyxoviridae); SSPE is a **late complication of a measles** infection that is not eliminated from the host. Immunization against measles is the only effective preventive tool.

Treatment

No specific therapy available.

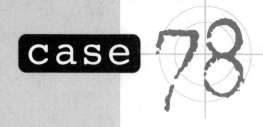

ID/CC A 5-year-old man presents with malaise, anorexia, fever, and a **pruritic rash on his scalp**, face, and trunk.

HPI He also complains of a headache. Six of his **classmates** recently missed school because of **similar symptoms**.

PE VS: fever (39°C). PE: skin lesions consist of **macules, papules, vesicles, pustules, and scabs,** all **present at same time,** predominantly over trunk, face, and scalp.

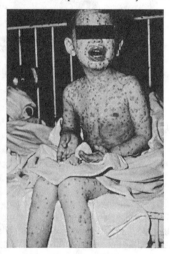

Figure 78-1. Macular, papular, vesicular, and pustular rash with scab formation.

Labs Multinucleated giant cells on scraping samples from vesicles. CBC: **leukopenia.**

Gross Pathology Macular, papular, vesicular, and pustular rash with scab formation; characteristically, all lesions present at same time **(vs. variola); lesions appear in crops** every 3 to 5 days; myocarditis and pneumonitis may be present.

Micro Pathology Intranuclear, acidophilic inclusion bodies (LIPSCHÜTZ BODIES) in epithelial cells with clear halo around them and multinucleated giant cells on histologic exam of skin lesions (on **Tzanck smear**).

155

case 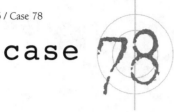78

Varicella (Chicken Pox)

Differential

Contact Dermatitis

Herpes Simplex

Impetigo

Urticaria

Discussion

A highly contagious dermotropic viral disease caused by VZV, a DNA herpesvirus, chickenpox is transmitted by respiratory aerosol or by direct contact. Complications include secondary bacterial infection of the skin and pneumonia; high-risk individuals may be protected passively with immunoglobulin and/or acyclovir. Vaccination of all children with a live attenuated vaccine is now recommended.

■ TABLE 78-1 SMALLPOX AND CHICKEN POX

	Smallpox	Chicken Pox
Fever	Occurs 2–4 days before rash onset	Occurs at the time of rash, if at all
Rash		
• **Distribution**	More lesions on the face and extremities; lesions on palms and soles	More lesions on the body; no lesions on palms and soles
• **Appearance**	Large, deep-seated vesicles or pustules in the same stage of development	Small, shallow vesicles in various stages of development
• **Course**	Lesions resolve over 14–21 days	Lesions resolve within 7–10 days
Mortality	10%–30%	Very uncommon

Treatment

Acetaminophen; antihistamines and calamine lotion; hygienic measures, including isolation.

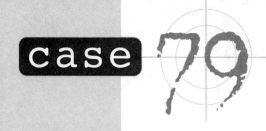

ID/CC A 24-year-old White, South American man develops sudden **high fever,** chills, generalized aches and pains, retro-orbital headache, nausea, and vomiting.

HPI He gradually improves, but the fever returns 4 days later along with a **yellowing of his skin and eyes** and an episode of fainting and abundant **coffee-ground emesis.**

PE VS: fever (39°C); hypotension (BP 90/60). PE: **jaundice;** petechiae on lower legs; swollen, bleeding gums; cardiomegaly; hepatomegaly.

Labs CBC: **leukopenia;** thrombocytopenia. UA: oliguria; **albuminuria;** hematuria.

Gross Pathology Normal-sized liver with yellowish hue and petechiae; pale, swollen kidneys.

Micro Pathology Characteristic **midzonal lobular necrosis** with sparing of central veins and portal triads; fatty accumulation and eosinophilic intracytoplasmic **Councilman bodies** on liver biopsy; hyperplasia of endothelial cells surrounding lymphoid follicles of spleen; **severe renal tubular damage** with epithelial fatty degeneration and necrosis.

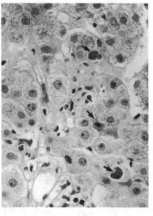

Figure 79-1. Councilman body *(arrow).*

VIROLOGY

157

case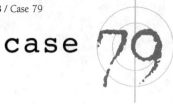

Yellow Fever

Differential

Acanthamoeba Infection
Relapsing Fever
Hemorrhagic Fever
Alcoholic Liver Disease

Discussion

Yellow fever is a viral hemorrhagic fever that is caused by a flavivirus transmitted by *Aedes* **mosquitoes;** it is preventable by a vaccine, which is required prior to travel to certain countries. It is associated with a mortality rate of 5%–10%, but most cases are self-limiting and mild. It is similar to malaria but does not recur.

■ TABLE 79-1 IMPORTANT HUMAN ARBOVIRUSES

Genus and Example	Main Disease	Primary Vector	Distribution
Togaviridae family			
Eastern equine encephalitis	Encephalitis	Mosquito	Eastern United States, Caribbean
Venezuelan equine encephalitis	Encephalitis	Mosquito	Central and South America
Ross River	Rash, arthritis	Mosquito	Australia
Many others	Fevers, arthritis, rash, encephalitis	Mosquito	Worldwide
Flaviviridae family			
West Nile	Encephalitis	Mosquito	Americas, Africa, Middle East, Europe
St. Louis encephalitis	Encephalitis	Mosquito	North America
Japanese encephalitis	Encephalitis	Mosquito	Asia, India, Australia
Dengue	Rash, hemorrhagic fever	Mosquito	Caribbean, South and Central America, Asia
Yellow fever	Hemorrhagic fever	Mosquito	Africa, South America
Tickborne encephalitis	Encephalitis	Tick	Russia, eastern and central Europe, Japan
Many others	Encephalitis	Mosquito, tick	Worldwide
Bunyaviridae family			
California	Encephalitis	Mosquito	North America
Rift Valley	Fever	Mosquito	Africa, Middle East
Sandfly fever	Fever	Sandfly	Mediterranean
Crimean-Congo hemorrhagic fever	Hermorrhagic fever	Tick, culicoid fly	Europe, Africa, Asia
Others	Fever	Mosquito	Worldwide

Treatment

Symptomatic; prevention with mosquito control and live viral vaccination.

ID/CC	A 38-year-old man receiving cytotoxic **chemotherapy** (immunosuppressed) for acute leukemia presents with **pleuritic chest pain,** hemoptysis, **fever,** and chills.
HPI	He also complains of dyspnea, tachypnea, and a **productive cough.**
PE	VS: fever. PE: severe respiratory distress; bilateral rales heard over lungs.
Labs	CBC: severe **neutropenia.** Negative blood and sputum culture for bacteria.
Imaging	CXR: necrotizing bronchopneumonia. CT, chest: ground-glass infiltrate with nodular densities (halo sign); wedge-shaped infiltrates.
Gross Pathology	**Necrotizing bronchopneumonia;** abscesses.
Micro Pathology	Lung biopsy identifies fungi with septate, acutely branching hyphae (visualized by silver stains); necrotizing inflammation; vascular thrombi with hyphae (due to **blood vessel invasion**).

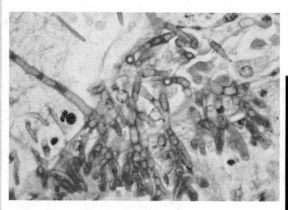

Figure 80-1. Septate, branching hyphae in tissue.

case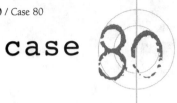

Aspergillosis

Differential

Asthma

Eosinophilic Pneumonia

Lung Abscess

Nocardiosis

Tuberculosis

Bacterial Pneumonia

Wegener Granulomatosis

Discussion

The most lethal form of infection, invasive aspergillosis, is seen primarily in severely immunocompromised individuals, i.e., patients with **AIDS**; patients with prolonged, **severe neutropenia** following cytotoxic chemotherapy; patients with **chronic granulomatous disease**; and patients receiving **glucocorticoids** and other **immunosuppressive drugs** (e.g., transplant recipients).

Breakout Point

Identification of Fungal Forms
Candida–Pseudohyphae
Aspergillosis–Septate, Hyphae branching at <45°
Mucor–Nonseptate, Hyphae branching at >90°
Blastomycosis–Broad-based budding
Paracoccidioidomycosis–Captain's Wheel Appearance

Treatment

IV amphotericin B or itraconazole.

case

ID/CC
A 50-year-old man presents to the ER with complaints of **recurrent,** sudden-onset, **severe breathlessness,** wheezing, fever, chills, and a **productive cough** (sometimes producing **brown bronchial casts**).

HPI
The patient has had steroid-dependent **chronic bronchial asthma** for many years and has no history of foreign travel or contact with a TB-infected patient. He has a history of **occasional hemoptysis.**

PE
VS: fever; marked tachycardia; severe tachypnea. PE: respiratory distress; central cyanosis; wheezing; rhonchi and coarse rales over both lung fields.

Labs
CBC: **eosinophilia.** Oxygen saturation low. Very high titers of specific **IgE antibodies against** *Aspergillus* present; sputum cultures positive for *Aspergillus*; **skin tests** to *Aspergillus* antigens **positive.** PFTs: obstructive picture.

Imaging
CXR: **segmental infiltrate** in upper lobes (these infiltrates are segmental because they correspond directly to the affected bronchi); **branching, fingerlike shadows** from mucoid impaction of dilated central bronchi (virtually **pathognomonic** of ABPA). CT, chest: evidence of **proximal bronchiectasis.**

case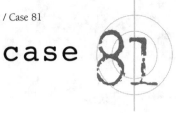

Aspergillosis—Allergic Bronchopulmonary

Differential

Asthma

Bronchiectasis

GERD

Primary Pulmonary Hypertension

Löffler Syndrome

Wegener Granulomatosis

Discussion

ABPA is a hypersensitivity disorder that primarily affects the central bronchi; immediate and Arthus-type hypersensitivity reactions are involved in its pathogenesis. The onset of the disease occurs most often in the fourth and fifth decades, and virtually all patients have long-standing atopic asthma. Untreated ABPA leads to proximal bronchiectasis.

Treatment

Oral corticosteroids or beclomethasone.

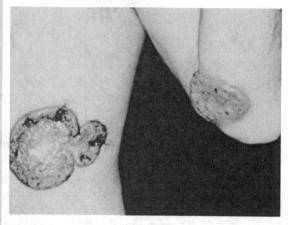
| ID/CC | A 32-year-old man is referred to a tertiary care center with **chronic pneumonia** and **warty lesions** on his left upper limb and chest wall. |

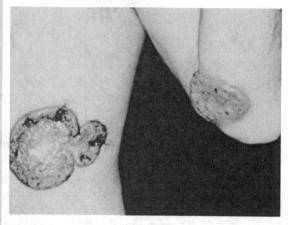

Figure 82-1. Progressive skin lesions with verrucous borders and an ulcerated center.

| HPI | The patient is from the **southeastern United States.** His skin lesions are nonpruritic and painless. He also complains of malaise, weight loss, night sweats, chest pain, breathlessness, and hoarseness. |

| PE | VS: fever; tachycardia; mild tachypnea. PE: **bilateral rales and rhonchi;** raised, **verrucous, and crusted lesions** with serpiginous border located on left upper extremity; small abscesses demonstrable when superficial crust was removed. |

| Labs | Sputum and pus from cutaneous lesions demonstrate **spherical cells** (8 to 15 mm in diameter) that have a **thick-walled, refractile double contour** and show unipolar (broad-based) budding. |

| Imaging | CXR: bilateral alveolar consolidations with air bronchograms. |

MYCOLOGY

case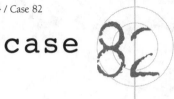

Blastomycosis

Differential

Actinomycosis
Aspergillosis
Cryptococcosis
Histoplasmosis
Sporotrichosis
Tuberculosis
Lung Cancer

Discussion

Blastomycosis is a systemic mycotic infection of humans and dogs that is characterized by suppuration and granulomatous lesions and is caused by the **dimorphic fungus *Blastomyces dermatitidis;*** the disease is **endemic in the southeastern and south-central portions of the United States,** and several pockets of infection extend north along the Mississippi and Ohio rivers into central Canada. Clinical disease most commonly involves the lungs (acquired by spore inhalation) and then, by hematogenous dissemination, the skin, the skeletal system, and the male GU tract. Infection cannot be passed from person to person.

Breakout Point

> ### Regional Distribution of Systemic Mycosis
>
> **Ohio/Mississippi River Valleys:** Histoplasmosis
> **Southwestern United States:** Coccidioidomycosis
> **Southeastern United States:** Blastomycosis

Treatment

Itraconazole is treatment of choice for mild to moderately severe cases; amphotericin B for life-threatening presentations.

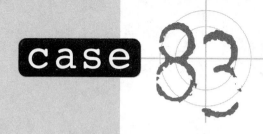

ID/CC A 49-year-old morbidly **obese, diabetic** woman presents with **pruritus in the skin folds** beneath her breasts.

HPI She admits to having this problem chronically, especially in the warm summer months when she perspires more heavily.

PE Superficially **denuded, beefy-red areas** beneath breasts with satellite vesicopustules and **whitish curd-like concretions** on surface.

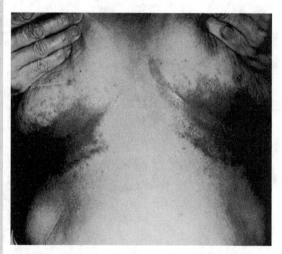

Figure 83-1. Beefy red lesions under the breasts.

Labs Clusters of **budding cells with pseudohyphae** seen under high-power lens after skin scales have been put in 10% KOH.

Gross Pathology Rash has whitish-creamy pseudomembrane that covers an erythematous surface.

Micro Pathology Yeast invades superficial layers of epithelium.

MYCOLOGY

case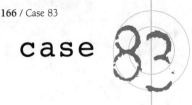

Candidiasis

Differential
Abscess
Streptococcal Infection
Staphylococcal Infection
Drug Eruption
Atopic Dermatitis

Discussion
Other superficial areas of infection include the oral mucosa (thrush), vaginal mucosa (vaginitis), and esophagus (GI candidiasis). Systemic invasive candidiasis may be seen with immunosuppression, in patients receiving **chronic broad-spectrum antibiotics,** in patients with AIDS, or in those receiving hyperalimentation.

Treatment
Keep affected areas dry; clotrimazole or other antifungal agents locally.

ID/CC A 19-year-old migrant worker from the **southwestern United States** is brought to the family doctor complaining of **cough, pleuritic chest pain, fever,** and malaise.

HPI He also complains of a backache and headache along with an **erythematous skin rash** (due to hypersensitivity reaction) in his lower limbs.

PE VS: fever; tachypnea. PE: central trachea; coarse, crepitant rales over both lung bases; tender, **erythematous nodules over shins** (ERYTHEMA NODOSUM); periarticular swelling of knees and ankles.

Labs **Dimorphic fungi** (hyphae in soil; spherules in body tissue); CBC/PBS: eosinophilia.

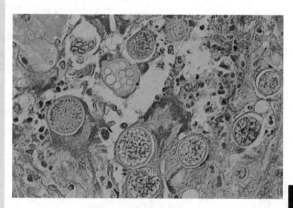

Figure 84-1. Spherule containing multiple endospores within lung tissue.

Imaging CXR: nodular infiltrates and thin-walled cavities in both lower lungs.

Gross Pathology **Caseating granulomas;** often subpleural and in lower lobes; necrosis and cavitation may also be present.

Micro Pathology Silver-stained tissue sections show spherules filled with endospores.

MYCOLOGY

case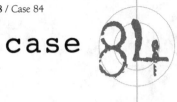

Coccidioidomycosis

Differential

Babesiosis

Erythema Multiforme

Staphylococcal Infection

Sarcodiosis

Lung Tumor

Discussion

Endemic in the southwestern United States, coccidioidomycosis is produced by *Coccidioides immitis* and is transmitted by **inhalation of arthrospores.** Systemic dissemination is frequent in Blacks as well as in immunosuppressed and pregnant patients. Meningitis or granulomatous lung disease may result, which may lead to death.

Treatment

Amphotericin B or itraconazole.

case 85

ID/CC	A 27-year-old White woman complains of **mouth ulcers, prolonged fever,** flulike symptoms, and increasing fatigue and weight loss over the past 2 months.
HPI	She recently moved from a large metropolitan area to a farm in **Ohio,** where she spent 1 week cleaning a **pigeons' loft.**
PE	VS: fever (38.5°C). PE: pallor; weight loss; enlarged liver and spleen; generalized lymphadenopathy; scattered sibilant rales over lung fields.
Labs	CBC/PBS: anemia; leukopenia. Small, budding fungus found **intracellularly in reticuloendothelial cells** (macrophages) on silver stain; elevated LDH; positive blood culture for dimorphic fungus.

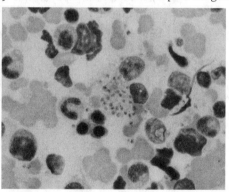

Figure 85-1. Highly characteristic image shows macrophage filled with 1-μm to 2-μm yeast cells.

Imaging	CXR: nonsegmental shifting pneumonic infiltrates; mediastinal adenopathy with popcorn calcifications; bilateral **hilar adenopathy.** CT, abdomen: splenic calcifications.
Micro Pathology	**Granulomas** with epithelioid cells, Langhans giant cells, and organisms within macrophages; in disseminated disease, organisms present in RES throughout body with proliferation.

169

MYCOLOGY

case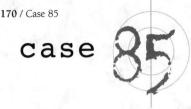

Histoplasmosis

Differential

Aspergillosis
Blastomycosis
Chlamydia Pneumonia
Sarcoidosis
Lung Tumor
Lymphoma

Discussion

Histoplasmosis is a systemic fungal infection some-times resembling TB that is caused by *Histoplasma capsulatum*, a dimorphic fungus. The yeast form is found intracellularly; the mold form is found in soil associated with **bird or bat feces.** Transmitted by inhalation of mold spores, it varies in intensity from asymptomatic to fulminant (in immunocompromised patients). The disease is most prevalent in the south-eastern, mid-Atlantic, and central regions of the United States.

Treatment

Itraconazole; amphotericin B.

case 86

ID/CC A 33-year-old HIV positive White man is brought into the ER by his mother because he complains of having a **persistent headache**.

HPI The patient's mother states that her son has been suffering for a long time from **headaches** and **stiff neck**, as well as from fever and chills.

PE VS: fever (39°C). PE: **severe nuchal rigidity;** lack of responsiveness to any command; positive **Kernig** and **Brudzinski** signs; diminished patellar and Achilles reflexes; clear lung sounds.

Labs LP: increased CSF pressure; variable pleocytosis (75 lymphocytes/mm³); elevated protein; decreased glucose. **Heavily encapsulated, nondimorphic spherical fungal cells revealed on India-ink staining;** polysaccharide capsular antigen detected on latex agglutination test; diagnosis confirmed by culture on Sabouraud medium.

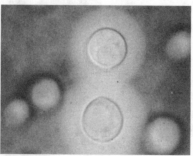

Figure 86-1. India-ink preparation shows halo effect around the yeast, caused by the large capsule.

Imaging CT/MR, brain: **multiple ring-enhancing lesions.**

Gross Pathology Granuloma and abscess formation, mainly at base of brain; CNS primarily affected; lungs affected less commonly.

Micro Pathology Abundant fungi in CSF and leptomeninges, with slight mononuclear inflammatory reaction; typical **nodular granulomatous meningitis** with exudate.

case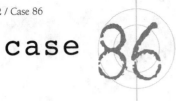

Meningitis—Cryptococcal

Differential
Toxoplasmosis
Aseptic Meningitis
CNS Vasculitis
Meningeal Carcinomatosis
Encephalitis
Bacterial Meningitis

Discussion
Once called torulosis, cryptococcosis is the most common cause of mycotic meningitis; it is acquired through the inhalation of dried **pigeon droppings** and is usually seen in **immunocompromised patients.**

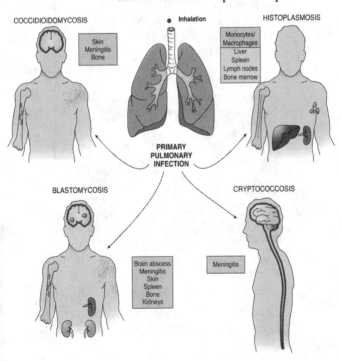

Figure 86-2. Systemic mycosis.

Treatment
Amphotericin B and 5-flucytosine; fluconazole.

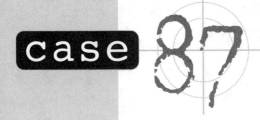

case 87

<table>
<tr><td>ID/CC</td><td>A 24-year-old White woman with IDDM is hospitalized for ketoacidosis following a night out drinking; on the fifth day she develops left periorbital swelling and a mucopurulent postnasal discharge that fails to respond to antibiotics.</td></tr>
</table>

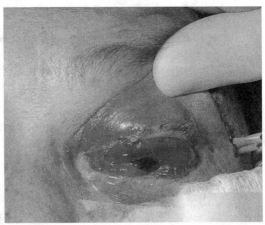

Figure 87-1. Periorbital edema, erythema, and chemosis.

HPI	She admits to irregular adherence to glucose control and insulin dosing.
PE	Left **periorbital** and paranasal **edema**; swelling of conjunctiva (CHEMOSIS); exophthalmos; **black ulceration of nasal mucosa; third CN palsy**.
Labs	**Large, irregular, nonseptate hyphae branching at wide (>90°) angles** on nasal culture.
Imaging	XR, plain: opacification of paranasal sinuses.
Gross Pathology	Necrotic destruction of paranasal sinuses and orbit, with dissemination to lung and brain.
Micro Pathology	Purulent arteritis with thrombi composed of hyphae; inflammation and necrosis with polymorphonuclear infiltrate.

173

MYCOLOGY

case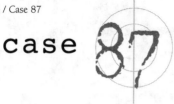

Mucormycosis

Differential

Cellulitis

Sinusitis

Nocardiosis

Actinomycosis

Nasopharyngeal Carcinoma

Discussion

Mucormycosis is a phycomycosis produced by *Mucor and Rhizopus* molds; it should be suspected in cases of antibiotic-resistant sinusitis, especially in the presence of underlying diabetes, burns, lymphoma, or leukemia.

Breakout Point

> *Mucor* and *Rhizopus* are unique in that they are fungi that cause disease in humans in their sexual phase.

Treatment

Amphotericin B; aggressive **surgical debridement**; prevent with tighter glucose control.

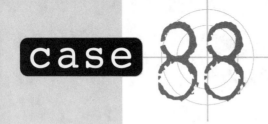

case 88

ID/CC A 30-year-old Black man presents with a nonpruritic **skin rash on the trunk, upper arm, and neck.**

HPI The patient is otherwise in excellent health.

PE Multiple **hypopigmented, scaling, confluent macules** seen on **trunk, upper arms, and neck;** no sensory loss demonstrated over areas of hypopigmentation; **Wood lamp** examination of skin macules displays a **pale-yellow to blue-white fluorescence.**

Labs Examination of KOH mounting of scales from lesions demonstrates the presence of short, thick, tangled hyphae with clusters of large, spherical budding yeast cells with characteristic **"spaghetti-and-meatballs"** appearance.

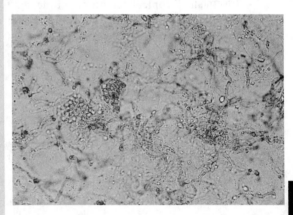

Figure 88-1. Short-branched hyphae and spores resembling spaghetti and meatballs.

case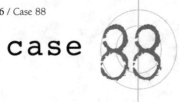

Pityriasis Versicolor

Differential

Pityriasis Alba

Seborrheic Dermatitis

Tinea Corporis

Vitiligo

Discussion

Pityriasis versicolor, which is common in young adults, is a relatively asymptomatic superficial skin infection caused by the lipophilic fungal organism **Pityrosporum orbiculare** (also termed *Malassezia furfur*). The lesions, which usually have a follicular origin, are small, hypopigmented-to-tan macules with a branlike scale; the macules are distributed predominantly on areas of the **upper trunk, neck,** and **shoulders.**

Treatment

Topical selenium sulfide; antifungal agents such as **miconazole** and **clotrimazole;** oral itraconazole in recalcitrant cases.

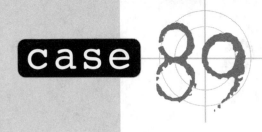
ID/CC A 32-year-old **HIV-positive man** presents with **progressively increasing dyspnea** over the past 3 weeks.

HPI He also complains of a **dry, painful cough**, marked **fatigue**, and a continuous **low-grade fever**. He has been noncompliant with cotrimoxazole prophylaxis.

PE VS: fever; marked **tachypnea**. PE: pallor; generalized lymphadenopathy; respiratory distress; **intercostal retraction**; mild central cyanosis; nasal flaring; coarse, crepitant rales auscultated at both lung bases.

Labs Cup-shaped organisms seen on **methenamine silver stain** of induced sputum or bronchoalveolar lavage; ELISA/Western blot positive for HIV. CBC: **leukopenia** with depressed CD4 cell count. **Serum LDH typically elevated.**

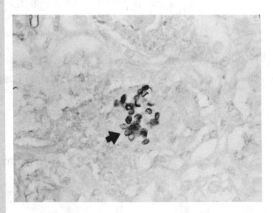

Figure 89-1. The 4-μm to 6-μm encysted cup or helmet-shaped organisms (*arrow*).

Imaging CXR: diffuse, bilaterally symmetrical **interstitial and alveolar infiltration** pattern, predominantly perihilar; no lymphadenopathy or effusion.

case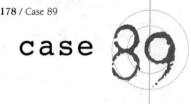

Pneumocystis carinii Pneumonia

Differential

Acute Respiratory Distress Syndrome

Mycoplasma Pneumonia

CMV Pneumonia

Mycobacterium Avium–Intracellular Infection

Bacterial Pneumonia

Viral Pneumonia

Tuberculosis

Discussion

Pneumocystis carinii pneumonia (PCP) is an opportunistic infection that causes interstitial pneumonia in many **immunocompromised** patients. Traditionally it has been classified as a protozoan; however, *P. carinii* ribosomal RNA indicates that the organism is **fungal**. It is seen in the upper lobes in patients receiving inhaled pentamidine prophylaxis. Treat HIV-positive patients prophylactically with TMP-SMX for *P. carinii* pneumonia if the CD4 count is <200.

Breakout Point

> ### Key Finding in *P. Carinii* Pneumonia
>
> ABGs that demonstrate **hypoxemia out of proportion to clinical findings.**

Treatment

IV **TMP-SMX;** alternative antimicrobials for patients sensitive to TMP-SMX include **pentamidine,** atovaquone, and clindamycin; steroids for severe disease.

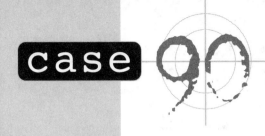

ID/CC A 37-year-old **gardener** complains of lumps with **red streaks** on his arm and swelling of the axillary lymph nodes.

HPI Two weeks ago, he **pricked his hand with a thorn** while pruning roses. A **nodule** then formed which subsequently **ulcerated** and filled with pus.

PE Nonpainful nodular lesion on dorsum of hand with ulcer formation and suppuration; **tender, palpable inflammation and hardening of lymph vessels** (LYMPHANGITIS); **swelling, inflammation, and suppuration of lymph nodes** (LYMPHADENITIS); nonulcerated satellite nodules along course of lymphatics.

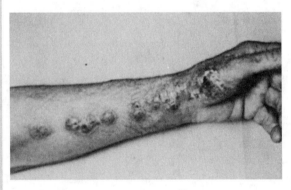

Figure 90-1. Chain of ulcerating nodules.

Labs **Cigar-shaped budding cells** visible in pus; diagnosis confirmed by culture of aspirate of nodule.

Gross Pathology **Nonpainful, soft, ulcerated nodule at inoculation site;** may extend to deep tissues and bone with osteitis and synovitis.

Micro Pathology Usually area of suppuration with polymorphonuclear infiltrate surrounded by granulomatous reaction of varied intensity with epithelioid and giant cell formation; chlamydospore asteroid bodies present.

MYCOLOGY

case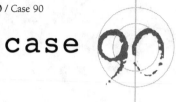

Sporotrichosis

Differential

Blastomycosis

Leishmaniasis

Paracoccidioidomycosis

Tularemia

Staphylococcal Infection

Discussion

Also called **"rose gardener's disease,"** sporotrichosis is a fungal infection caused by *Sporothrix schenckii*, a dimorphic fungus that lives on vegetation. It is typically transmitted by a thorn prick and causes localized infection with few systemic manifestations.

Treatment

Itraconazole; amphotericin B for meningeal or disseminated infection.

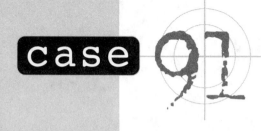

case 91

ID/CC A 30-year-old man presents with a bilateral **red pruritic** skin **eruption** in the **groin** area.

PE Bilateral, **circular papulosquamous skin eruption** on erythematous base with **active,** advancing **peripheral (serpiginous) border** over scrotum and perineum.

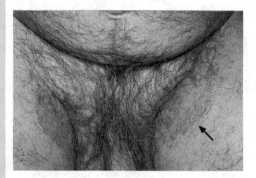

Figure 91-1. Note *(arrow)* the scalloped shape with an "active border."

Labs Microscopic examination reveals long septate **hyphae on KOH** skin scrapings.

case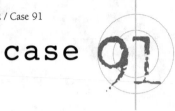

Tinea Cruris (Ringworm/Jock Itch)

Differential
Cutaneous Candidiasis
Impetigo
Nummular Dermatitis
Pityriasis Rosea
Tinea Versicolor
Psoriasis

Discussion
Tinea cruris and tinea corporis (COMMON RINGWORM) occur sporadically; *Trichophyton rubrum* is the most common cause. The inflammatory form, which is usually localized to the limbs, chest, or back, is commonly caused by *Microsporum canis* or *Trichophyton mentagrophytes*. Ringworm of the scalp, known as tinea capitis, is commonly seen in children and is caused by *Trichophyton tonsurans*.

Breakout Point

Tinea and Locations
Tinea capitus—head
Tinea corpus—body
Tinea cruris—groin (jock itch)
Tinea pedis—foot (athlete's foot)
Tinea unginum—nail bed

Treatment
Topical antifungal agents (clotrimazole, miconazole); systemic therapy with oral griseofulvin, terbinafine, ketoconazole, or itraconazole in extensive or resistant cases.

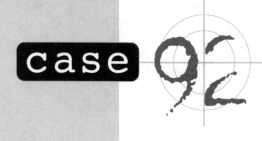

case 92

ID/CC A 35-year-old man complains of **cough** productive of mucopurulent sputum and of **breathlessness**.

HPI Before the onset of these symptoms, he had a sore throat with hoarseness. He has no history of hemoptysis, sharp chest pain, or high-grade fever.

PE Crepitations heard over left lung base.

Labs CBC: normal leukocyte count. Sputum exam revealed no **bacterial organism;** positive indirect microimmunofluorescence test for *Chlamydia pneumoniae* **antibodies.**

Imaging CXR: left lower lobe subsegmental infiltrate with interstitial pattern.

case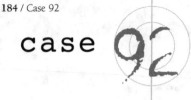

Chlamydia Pneumonia

Differential

Influenza

Legionnaire's Disease

Mycoplasma Pneumonia

Psittacosis

Q Fever

Tuberculosis

Discussion

Chlamydia pneumoniae causes mild lower respiratory infection in young adults, but older adults suffer more serious disease. It is transmitted by respiratory droplets.

Treatment

Doxycycline is the drug of choice; alternatively, **erythromycin** may be used.

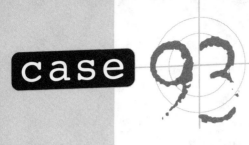

case 93

ID/CC	An 8-year-old boy who recently emigrated from India presents with **bilateral eye irritation** and **photophobia.**
HPI	He reports **recurrent episodes** of similar eye irritation and redness **in the past.**
PE	Conjunctival congestion; **multiple (>5) follicles,** each at least 0.5 mm in diameter, seen **in upper tarsal conjunctiva;** inflammatory thickening of tarsal conjunctiva; new vessels (PANNUS) seen in cornea at superior limbus; **punctate keratitis.**

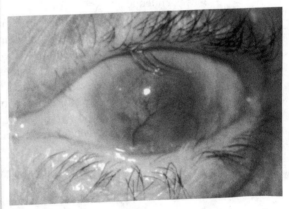

Figure 93-1. Typical eye findings.

Labs	Cell culture grows **elementary bodies.**
Micro Pathology	Histologically there is lymphocytic infiltration involving the whole adenoid layer of parts of the conjunctiva; special aggregations of lymphocytes form **follicles** that tend to show necrosis and certain large multinucleated cells (LEBER CELLS).

case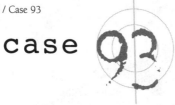

Chlamydia Trachomatis

Differential

Conjunctivitis
Reiter Syndrome
Sicca Syndrome
Corneal Abrasion
Uveitis

Discussion

Chlamydia trachomatis causes a variety of ocular diseases, including **neonatal inclusion conjunctivitis, sporadic inclusion conjunctivitis in adults, and sporadic as well as endemic trachoma;** trachoma is endemic in North Africa, in the Middle East, and among the Native American population of the southwestern United States. In endemic areas, trachoma is transmitted from eye to hand to eye, especially among young children in regions where standards of cleanliness are poor. Sporadic trachoma infection in nonendemic areas as well as sporadic inclusion conjunctivitis in adults results from transmission of the agent from the genital tract to the eye.

Breakout Point

> Trachoma is the leading cause of blindness worldwide.

Treatment

Topical **tetracycline** or erythromycin with systemic **tetracycline/doxycycline/erythromycin** for possible extraocular infection (GI or nasopharyngeal); prophylaxis of family contacts with topical tetracycline.

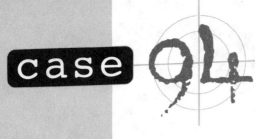

ID/CC A 30-year-old man from **Texas** presents with **fever and a skin rash** that began about 2 weeks ago.

HPI The onset was gradual, with prodromal symptoms of headache, malaise, backache, and chills. These symptoms were followed by shaking chills, fever, and a more severe headache accompanied by nausea and vomiting. A remittent pattern of fever accompanied by tachycardia continued for 10 to 12 days, with the **rash appearing around the fifth day of fever.** The patient **worked at a rat-infested food-storage depot** this summer.

PE VS: fever. PE: discrete, irregular pink **maculopapular rash** seen in axillae and on trunk, thighs, and upper arms; face, palms, and soles only sparsely involved; mild splenomegaly noted.

Labs The **Weil-Felix** agglutination reaction for *Proteus* strain **OX-19 was positive;** complement-fixing antibodies to the typhus group antigen were demonstrated.

case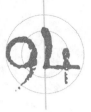

Endemic Typhus

Differential

Epidemic Typhus

Anthrax

Ehrlichiosis

Leptospirosis

Rocky Mountain Spotted Fever

Tularemia

Discussion

Murine typhus is a natural infection of rats and mice by *Rickettsia typhi*; **spread of infection to humans by the rat flea** is incidental and occurs when feces from infected fleas are scratched into the lesion. Cases can occur year-round; however, most occur during the summer months, primarily in southern Texas and California.

■ TABLE 94-1 RICKETTSIAL INFECTIONS

Disease	Organism	Distribution	Transmission
	Spotted-fever Group		
Rocky Mountain spotted fever	*Rickettsia rickettsii*	Americas	Ticks
Queensland tick fever	*Rickettsia australis*	Australia	Ticks
Boutonneuse fever, Kenya tick fever	*Rickettsia conorii*	Mediterranean, Africa, India	Ticks
Siberian tick fever	*Rickettsia sibirica*	Siberia, Mongolia	Ticks
Rickettsialpox	*Rickettsia akari*	United States, Russia, Central Asia, Korea, Africa	Mites
	Typhus group		
Louse-borne typhus (epidemic typhus)	*Rickettsia prowazekii*	Latin America, Africa, Asia	Lice
Murine typhus (endemic typhus)	*Rickettsia typhi*	Worldwide	Fleas
Scrub typhus	*Rickettsia tsutsugamushi*	South Pacific, Asia	Mites
Q fever	*Coxiella burnetti*	Worldwide	Inhalation

Treatment

Antibiotic treatment with **doxycycline** (**chloramphenicol** is used as an alternative).

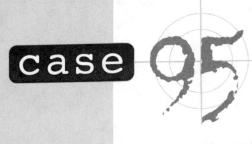

case 95

ID/CC	A 28-year-old Guatemalan man is brought to the hospital complaining of **severe headache**, photophobia, and fever over the past 2 weeks.
HPI	As a political dissident, he spent 4 months in a **refugee camp** in southern Mexico before entering the United States.
PE	VS: fever (40°C). PE: papilledema and delirium; bilateral swelling of parotid glands 1 week later; toxic facies; maculopapular **rash** on trunk and extremities; **face, palms, and soles spared**; mild splenomegaly.

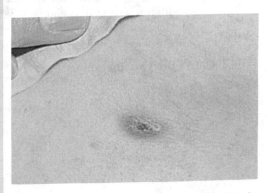

Figure 95-1. Erythematous macule with central black eschar.

Labs	**Positive Weil-Felix reaction** to OX-19 strains of *Proteus*; UA: proteinuria; microscopic hematuria.
Gross Pathology	Myocarditis and pneumonia may be present; cerebral edema; maculopapular rash.
Micro Pathology	**Zenker degeneration of striated muscle**; thrombosis and endothelial proliferation of capillaries with abundant rickettsiae and perivascular cuffing; accumulation of lymphocytes.

189

case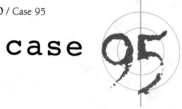

Epidemic Typhus

Differential	Endemic Typhus
	Anthrax
	Ehrlichiosis
	Leptospirosis
	Rocky Mountain Spotted Fever
	Tularemia
Discussion	Epidemic typhus is a febrile illness caused by *Rickettsia prowazekii,* a gram-negative, nonmotile, obligate intracellular parasite; it is transmitted via **body lice** and is associated with **war, famine,** and **crowded living conditions.** The rash should be differentiated from Rocky Mountain spotted fever, which starts peripherally on the wrists and ankles and also includes the palms and soles.
Treatment	**Doxycycline;** chloramphenicol.

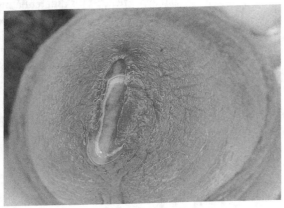

case 96

ID/CC	A **28-year-old man** comes to the ER with gradually worsening and now severe **scrotal swelling** and pain radiating to the inguinal area.
HPI	The patient has no significant medical history. He reports pain on urination (due to concomitant urethritis) and notes that he is sexually active with multiple partners. He also notes that the pain is greater on standing and walking and is relieved by rest and elevation of the legs.

Figure 96-1. Purulent urethral discharge.

PE	VS: normal. PE: **scrotal edema** and erythema; **right epididymis enlarged and tender**; induration present; **elevation** of scrotal contents **relieves pain** (PREHN SIGN).
Labs	UA: pyuria. Culture negative.
Imaging	US: hypoechoic, enlarged epididymis with hypervascularity.
Gross Pathology	Nonspecific inflammation characterized by congestion and edema.
Micro Pathology	Early stage of the infection is limited to the interstitial connective tissue with white cell infiltration.

191

case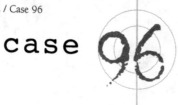

Epididymitis

Differential

Hydrocele

Scrotal Trauma

Testicular Seminoma

Testicular Torsion

Testicular Trauma

Discussion

Differentiate epididymitis from testicular torsion and tumor (scrotal ultrasonography or isotopic flow study may be needed for differentiating). Transmitted sexually in young adults and most often **caused by *Chlamydia trachomatis* subtypes D through K** and *Neisseria gonorrhoeae*. In those older than 40, *Escherichia coli* and *Pseudomonas* cause most infections. If associated with rectal intercourse, it may be due to *Enterobacteriaceae*.

Treatment

Antibiotics like doxycycline, minocycline for chlamydia. Course of ofloxacin covers all possibilities of causative organisms.

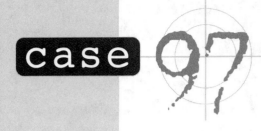

ID/CC A 25-year-old man complains of swollen, **tender masses in his groin** and very painful **genital ulcers** of 1 week's duration.

HPI The patient admits to having had **unprotected sex** with multiple partners.

PE **Swollen,** erythematous, tender **inguinal nodes,** usually bilateral, with draining sinuses (INGUINAL ADENITIS, BUBOES); multiple small genital lesions.

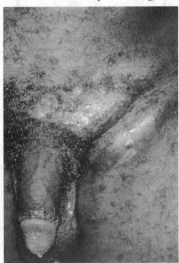

Figure 97-1. Inguinal pseudobubo.

Labs Inguinal node biopsy diagnostic; **positive complement fixation test; positive immunofluorescence test.**

Gross Pathology Primary lesion is ulcerated nodule; gives rise to **inguinal bubo,** an enlarged lymph node sometimes characterized by fistulous tract formation; balanitis, phimosis, and rectal involvement with stricture may also be present.

Micro Pathology Neutrophilic infiltration of primary lesion with areas of necrosis; lymphoid hyperplasia of lymph nodes with foci of macrophage accumulation; abscess formation with fibrosis.

193

case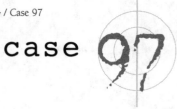

Lymphogranuloma Venereum

Differential	Plaque Hodgkin Disease Non-Hodgkin Lymphoma Inflammatory Proctocolitis Mycobacterial Infection
Discussion	Lymphogranuloma venereum is an STD that is due to ***Chlamydia trachomatis* (L1, L2, L3).** Counseling should be given about other STDs (e.g., AIDS, syphilis, gonorrhea).
Treatment	**Doxycycline;** erythromycin.

case 98

ID/CC A 35-year-old man presents with high **fever**, malaise, headache, and a **hacking cough productive** of a small amount of mucoid sputum.

HPI He has two **pet parrots** at home who have recently shown **signs of illness**.

PE VS: fever; **bradycardia**. PE: auscultation of chest reveals **crepitant rales** over both lower lung fields; **splenomegaly** with mild hepatomegaly noted; multiple erythematous macules seen on face (HORDER SPOTS).

Labs Definitive diagnosis is in progress.

Imaging CXR, PA: **interstitial** patchy, bilateral **infiltrates**.

Gross Pathology Principal lesions found in lungs, liver, and spleen.

Micro Pathology Pulmonary lesion is an **interstitial pneumonitis**; mononuclear cells with ballooned cytoplasm containing inclusion bodies are observed. In the liver, focal necrosis of hepatocyte occurs along with Kupffer cell hyperplasia.

case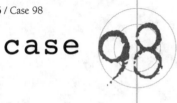

Psittacosis

Differential

Chlamydia Pneumonia
Legionnaire's Disease
Q Fever
Tularemia
Mycobacterial Infection
Bacterial Pneumonia

Discussion

Psittacosis is an acute infection caused by *Chlamydia psittaci*; it is characterized primarily by pneumonitis and systemic manifestations and is **transmitted** to humans by a variety of avian species, **principally psittacine birds (parrots, parakeets).** A history of contact with birds, particularly sick birds, or of employment in a pet shop or in the poultry industry provides a clue to the diagnosis of psittacosis in a patient with pneumonia, especially if bradycardia and splenomegaly are also present.

Treatment

Doxycycline; macrolides such as azithromycin are effective alternatives.

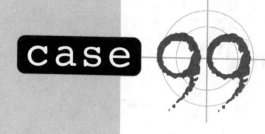

ID/CC	A 30-year-old **dairy-farm worker** presents with complaints of **fever, headache, cough, pleuritic chest pain,** and malaise.
HPI	His work at the dairy involves **milking cows** and **looking after parturient cattle.**
PE	VS: fever; tachypnea. PE: mild icterus; bilateral **crackles** on chest auscultation.
Labs	CBC: normal WBC count. Mild elevation of serum bilirubin and liver enzymes; **negative Weil-Felix reaction.**
Imaging	CXR: right upper lobe **rounded opacity** that increased in size over a few days and cleared completely with treatment.

case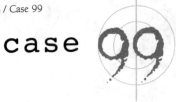

Q Fever

Differential

Chronic Fatigue Syndrome
Influenza
Atypical Pneumonia
Infective Endocarditis
Fever of Unknown Origin
Meningitis

Discussion

Q fever is caused by the rickettsia-like organism *Coxiella burnetii* and produces the clinical picture of primary atypical pneumonia. Q fever differs from the other human rickettsioses in that rash is absent and **transmission** is usually **by the airborne route.** *C. burnetii* localizes in the **mammary glands and uterus of pregnant cattle**, sheep, and goats, in which infection is mild or inapparent; **infected placentas, postpartum discharges, and the feces of these animals** are the **principal sources of contaminated material** in the environment. Humans acquire Q fever by inhaling aerosolized particles from such substances; particularly **at risk** are **dairy and slaughterhouse workers.**

Treatment

Doxycycline is the first-line agent of therapy; fluoroquinolones and macrolides are effective alternatives (erythromycin can also be used).

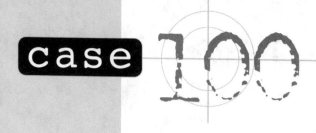

case 100

ID/CC A 6-year-old boy presents with fever, intense headache, myalgia, dry cough, and a **rash that began peripherally** (on his wrists and ankles) but now involves the entire body, **including the palms and soles.**

HPI The child lives in North Carolina and indicates that he was **bitten by an insect** a few weeks ago while playing in the woods near his home.

PE VS: fever. PE: lethargy; ill appearance; **petechial rash** all over body, including palms and soles.

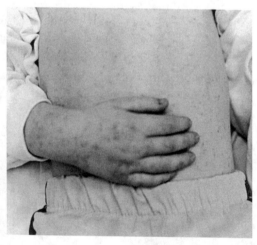

Figure 100-1. Petechial rash on the trunk and hands.

Labs CBC: thrombocytopenia; prolonged bleeding and clotting time. Positive Hess capillary test (RUMPEL-LEEDE PHENOMENON). UA: proteinuria; hematuria.

Gross Pathology Hemorrhagic necrosis in brain and kidneys; nodular formation in glia.

Micro Pathology Inflammatory lymphocytic and plasma cell perivascular infiltration; endothelial edema with abundant rickettsiae; microthrombus formation **with necrotic vasculitis.**

case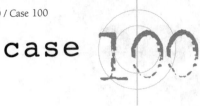

Rocky Mountain Spotted Fever

Differential	Lyme Disease
	Disseminated Gonococcal Disease
	Drug Reaction
	Syphilis
	Measles
	HFMD
Discussion	*Rickettsia rickettsii* is the causative organism of Rocky Mountain spotted fever; *Dermacentor*, **a wood tick, is the vector.** The organism's tropism for endothelial cells results in vasculitis, edema, thrombosis, and ischemia. Ironically, Rocky Mountain spotted fever is endemic to the East Coast of the United States.
Treatment	**Doxycycline** or **chloramphenicol.**

questions

1. A 2-year-old child is brought to the pediatrician for his fourth case of sore throat in the last 6 months. Once again, the boy tests positive for strep throat. Other than an extremely fair complexion he appears normal. Analysis of his PBS reveals neutrophils with large lysosomes. A referral is made to an immunology clinic for concern of Chediak-Hagashi syndrome. Which of the following defects is present in such patients?

   A. A deficiency of C1 esterase inhibitor
   B. A selective deficiency of IgA
   C. Deficiency of Burton tyrosine kinase
   D. A defect in the polymerization of microtubules
   E. A defect in the β subunit of integrin

2. An 18-month-old boy has had several repeated infections since the age of 6 months. These infections have resulted in numerous hospitalizations for administration of IV antibiotics. As well, the child has had several enlarged lymph nodes and significant hepatosplenomegaly. His CBC is within normal limits, however, more thorough investigation of his WBC count shows a lack of normal respiratory burst, as demonstrated with nitroblue tetrazolium. Which of the following diseases is most likely in this child?

   A. Chronic granulomatous disease
   B. Wiskott-Aldrich syndrome
   C. Ataxia telangiectasia
   D. DiGeorge syndrome
   E. SCID

3. A 17-year-old female is referred to a gastroenterologist with persistent bloody diarrhea. She has no family history of inflammatory bowel disease. She admits to traveling to Mexico for her high school graduation and has really not felt well since returning 3 months ago. A colonoscopy is performed, demonstrating colonic mucosal ulceration. Biopsy reveals "flask-shaped" ulcers with trophozoites at the base. Which of the following is the most likely?

   A. *Giardia lamblia*
   B. Hepatitis A
   C. *Entamoeba histolytica*
   D. CMV
   E. *Cryptosporidium parvum*

4. A 27-year-old male who recently immigrated to the United States from Venezuela is seen in a community clinic with complaints of difficulty swallowing. A barium swallow study demonstrates that he has a significantly dilated proximal esophagus (megaesophagus) with significant narrowing at the gastroesophageal junction. An EGD with biopsy demonstrates destruction of the myenteric plexus by parasites. A tentative diagnosis of Chagas disease is rendered. Which of the following is the vector for the causative agent?

   A. Sandfly
   B. Dermacentor tick
   C. Anopheles mosquito
   D. Ixodes tick
   E. Reduviid bug

5. While on a tropical medicine rotation, a fourth-year medical student is stationed in a refugee camp. A 42-year-old male visits the clinic complaining of itching and loss of vision. The man's home, a makeshift cabin, is within a hundred yards of the river that runs through the camp. A thorough ophthalmologic exam demonstrates the presence of microfilaria in the eye. He is immediately started on ivermectin to treat which of the following?

   A. *Diphyllobothrium latum*
   B. *Onchocerca volvulus*
   C. *Ancylostoma duodenale*
   D. *Toxocara canis*
   E. *Trypanosoma brucei*

6. A 56-year-old man presents to the ER with complaints of RUQ abdominal pain. His liver enzymes are elevated, as is his bilirubin. His CBC is mildly elevated but with dramatic elevation of his eosinophil count. A CT scan demonstrates multiple large septated liver cysts. Upon obtaining further history, you learned he returned from a 2-month stay on a cousin's sheep range in New Zealand. Infectious disease is corrected regarding the possibility of hydatid disease. This disorder results from infection with which organism?

   A. *Taenia solium*
   B. *Naegleria fowleri*
   C. *Echinococcus granulosis*
   D. *Trichinella spiralis*
   E. *Loa loa*

7. A 22-year-old Peace Corps volunteer returns to the United States after a 6-month project in Jordan. As she was a social science major in college, she was assigned to help construct irrigation trenches on arid land to convert it to farmland. She spent many days wading knee high in irrigation water. She now complains of intensely pruritic skin eruptions and blood in her urine. A urine sample demonstrates ellipsoid eggs with a terminal spine suspicious for *Schistosoma haematobium*. Which of the following is a potential complication of this disease?

   A. Portal hypertension
   B. Transitional cell carcinoma of the bladder
   C. Squamous cell carcinoma of the bladder
   D. Maltoma of the stomach
   E. Cholangiocarcinoma

8. A 37-year-old patient with AIDS presents to the ER with complaints of headache and malaise. His CD4 count is 85 and his LP is negative for WBCs, bacteria, or organisms seen by India-ink staining. In addition, his glucose in the CSF is normal, as is the protein level. A CT scan of the head demonstrates a ring-enhancing mass. Given the likely presence of protozoal infection, which of the following represents the most likely source of infection?

   A. Contact with infected canine feces
   B. Direct person-to-person contact
   C. Consumption of contaminated unchlorinated water
   D. Consumption of raw meat
   E. Exposure to contaminated pigeon droppings

9. An 8-year-old child is brought to the pediatrician with complaints of "pink eye" in both eyes. It began 2 days ago after a school picnic where the children were taken to the community swimming pool. Several of the other children have stayed home from school. This child initially had one "red eye" that was itchy and now both eyes are involved. Of the following, which is the most likely pathogen?

   A. Adenovirus
   B. CMV
   C. HSV
   D. *Neisseria gonorrhea*
   E. *Chlamydia trachomatis*

10. A 14-year-old boy is brought to the family physician with complaints of high-grade fevers, myalgias, and headaches. He tells the physician that he recently returned from Boy Scout Jamboree in western Montana over the summer. He was not diligent with the use of repellent and he often went hiking without socks. A battery of tests suggests he has Colorado tick fever. Which of the following likely transferred this reovirus to the patient?

   A. *Wuchereria bancrofti*
   B. A rodent
   C. The *Culex* mosquito
   D. The *Dermacentor* tick
   E. An infected bat

11. A 4-year-old child is referred to a dermatologist for developing fatigue and a rash. The rash initially involved the face and started with a "slapped-cheek" appearance. Over the last few days the rash has progressed to involve the trunk and limbs. The boy also complains of pain in his joints. He has a low-grade fever. He does have a known family history of hereditary spherocytosis. His RBC count returns drastically decreased. The virus that underlies his illness is likely which of these?

   A. Unenveloped RNA virus
   B. Enveloped RNA virus
   C. A single-stranded unenveloped DNA virus
   D. A double-stranded enveloped DNA virus
   E. A retrovirus

12. An 18-year-old male presents to his family physician with "yellow eyes" and skin. He notes having episodes of diarrhea soon after returning from Mexico for a high school graduation trip. He admits to taking day trips to the country to "experience real life in Mexico." He also admits to eating and drinking food of "unquestionable cleanliness." His transaminases and bilirubin return elevated and he has IgM antibodies to HAV. What is the likely consequence of HAV infection?

   A. Complete resolution without sequela
   B. Development of fulminant hepatitis
   C. Resolution, but he will become a chronic carrier
   D. Development of cirrhosis
   E. Development of hepatocellular carcinoma

13. A 19-year-old volunteer at a blood bank notes that he thinks one of the sharps containers broke. In his haste to clean up, he reports that a needle used to draw blood stuck his hand. He was subsequently referred to the employee health section when his supervisor learned 1 week later that the incident occurred. The patient thinks that he received a hepatitis B vaccination at birth. Which of the following would be the result of his hepatitis panel, if indeed he was vaccinated?

A. HBsAg(-), anti-HBs(-), anti-HBc(-), anti-HBe(-), HBeAg(-)
B. HBsAg(-), anti-HBs(+), anti-HBc(-), anti-HBe(-), HBeAg(-)
C. HBsAg(-), anti-HBs(+), anti-HBc(+), anti-HBe(+), HBeAg(-)
D. HBsAg(+), anti-HBs(-), anti-HBc(+), anti-HBe(-), HBeAg(+)
E. HBsAg(+), anti-HBs(-), anti-HBc(+), anti-HBe(+), HBeAg(-)

14. A 75-year-old female is being treated for CLL. She now complains of a painful vesicular rash around her left eye. A Tzank smear, prepared from a grouping of vesicles, demonstrates acatholytic cells. She tells you she remembers having chicken pox long ago. She also tells you that in college she had the "kissing disease." Her current condition is likely due to which herpes virus?

A. HSV
B. CMV
C. EBV
D. VZV
E. KSHV

15. A 22-year-old male returns with a church group from spending the summer in eastern Europe. While there, he was helping a village rebuild after a devastating mudslide. He now complains of bilateral facial swelling as well as pain in his scrotum. While at the physician's office, an EIA is prepared. Results a week later show a fourfold increase in mumps antibodies. Which of the following is a long-term complication of the infection?

A. DIC
B. Nasopharyngeal Carcinoma
C. Burkitt Lymphoma
D. Subacute Sclerosing Panencephalitis
E. Sterility

16. While on a medical mission in India, an infectious disease specialist is brought to see a young boy, who has been bitten by a stray dog. The boy has developed fever and convulsions, and complains of numbness of the leg on which he was bitten. The stray dog is captured and its brain is sent for analysis. The boy is given postexposure HRIG. If the dog is truly infected, which of the following would describe the virions seen by electron microscopy?

   A. Bullet shaped
   B. Filamentous
   C. Icosahedral
   D. Brick shaped
   E. Safety-pin shaped

17. A 3-year-old male is brought to the ER by his mother, who says he has had severe runny diarrhea for a day. She notes many children in his day care also have had diarrhea. On exam, the child appears fussy and has poor skin turgor. The mother notes that there have been numerous fluid bowel movements, though there has been no blood in the stools. Which of the following is the likely etiologic agent?

   A. *Campylobacter jejuni*
   B. *Cryptosporidium parvum*
   C. Norwalk virus
   D. *Trichuris trichiura*
   E. Rotavirus

18. A 10-year-old child died of a long and progressively deteriorating condition. During his last months, he developed myoclonic seizures, extrapyrimidal signs, and personality changes. An autopsy is performed, and encephalitis involving both the white and gray matter with marked lymphocytic infiltration is noted. A diagnosis of SSPE is suspected. Which of the following is likely associated with this condition?

   A. Prions
   B. A defective measles M protein
   C. Congenital infection with rubella
   D. LCM infection
   E. Hepatitis D infection

19. A 23-year-old veterinary technician presents to the family physician with a fever, headache, malaise, arthralgias, and a dry cough. She denies any recent sick contacts. However, she admits that she worked weekends at the local pet store. Further questioning reveals that she often spends time in the section of the store that displays the parrots and parakeets. Which of the following organisms is likely to have caused her symptoms?

    A. *Rickettsia ricketsii*
    B. *Coxiella burnetti*
    C. *Rickettsia prowazeki*
    D. *Chlamydia psittaci*
    E. *Chlamydia trachomatis*

20. A 37-year-old female with poorly controlled diabetes mellitus presents in ketoacidosis to the ER. She complains of a severe frontal headache with vision changes. A CT scan of the head and sinuses reveals destruction of the sinus with extension of an abscess into the brain parenchyma. A biopsy is taken through the sphenoid sinus and mucomyosis is suspected. Which of the following would be demonstrated upon appropriate staining of the involved organism?

    A. Germ-tube formation
    B. Broad-based budding
    C. Septate hyphae branching at acute angles
    D. Nonseptate hyphae branching at greater than 90° angles
    E. "Spaghetti-and-meatballs" appearance

answers

1-D

A. Deficiency of C1 esterase inhibitor [incorrect] leads to a disorder known as hereditary angioedema. This autosomal-dominant disorder can result in life-threatening laryngeal edema.

B. The most common immunologic defect in the western world is selective IgA deficiency [incorrect]. The symptoms are often subtle, manifesting as recurrent sinopulmonary infections.

C. Deficiency of Burton tyrosine kinase [incorrect] results in Burton agammaglobulinemia. This disorder results from a virtual absence of all immunoglobulin subclasses, with senous, repeat bacterial infections around the time that maternally transplacentally transferred antibodies are lost.

D. Chediak-Hagashi syndrome results from a defect in the polymerization of microtubules [correct]. The result is defects in neutrophil degranulation with defective fusion of lysosomes, with phagosomes resulting in giant lysosomes. Patients with defective neutrophil killing suffer from recurrent infection from pyogenic organisms like *Streptococcus* and *Staphylococcus*.

E. Leukocyte adhesion deficiency I results from an autosomal recessive defect in the β subunit of integrins [incorrect]. This results in defects in WBC adhesion and migration, with recurrent soft tissue infections.

2-A

A. Patients with chronic granulomatous disease [correct] have defects in the formation of superoxide, the most important molecule in killing phagocytosed bacteria. The disease is most often due to an X-linked mutation in the gene for cytochrome oxidase. Patients are often treated with γ interferon.

B. Wiskott-Aldrich syndrome [incorrect] is due to an X-linked defect of the WASP gene. The typical presentation is that of a triad of eczema, thrombocytopenia, and recurrent bacterial infections.

C. Repair of recombining gene segments during the development of T cells and antibodies requires the gene product of the ataxia telangiectasia (AT) gene [incorrect]. Patients with AT have defective immune responses as well as increased likelihood of malignancy, vascular dilations (telangiectasia), and a staggering gait.

D. Defects in the migration of neural crest cells into the third and fourth pharyngeal pouches result in DiGeorge syndrome [incorrect]. These patients present with cardiac abnormalities, abnormal facies, thymic hypoplasia, hypocalcemia, and congenital cardiac disease.

E. Most often due to X-linked mutations in the adenosine deaminase gene, important in the purine salvage pathway, patients with SCID [incorrect] have severe defects in T-cell and B-cell development. Without an effective immune system, these patients require enzyme supplementation, bone marrow transplantation, or even gene therapy.

3-C

A. The most common protozoal disease in the United States is due to *Giardia lamblia* [incorrect]. However, giardiasis does not cause bloody diarrhea and does not invade the intestinal mucosa.

B. Hepatitis A [incorrect] is an enterovirus and infection that can be associated with gastroenteritis. However, once again there would be no bloody diarrhea, and it would likely be characterized by jaundice and increased transaminases.

C. *Entamoeba histolytica* [correct] causes bloody diarrhea because of invasion of the organism into the colonic mucosa. Once the organism hits the muscularis, it tunnels laterally, thus forming the flask-shaped ulcer. It is often acquired from contaminated water.

D. CMV [incorrect] can cause a severe life-threatening colitis in immunocompromised individuals. The characteristic histologic appearance of CMV-infected cells are the formation of cells with a large "owl's eye" nucleus.

E. Often associated with AIDS or immunocompetent individuals in large outbreaks due to contaminated water, Cryptosporidium [incorrect] infection causes a profuse, non bloody, watery diarrhea. Acid-fast staining of the stool often detects such organisms.

4-E

A. The sandfly [incorrect] is the vector for the parasitic organism Leishmania. Leishmaniasis causes a spectrum of clinical syndromes ranging from self-resolving cutaneous ulcers to fatal disseminated disease.

B. Rocky Mountain spotted fever (RMSF) is caused by the obligate intracellular organism, *Rickettsia rickettsii*. RMSF causes a potentially fatal vasculitis with head, fever, and a rash. It is transmitted by the Dermacentor tick [incorrect].

C. Malaria, is a hemolytic febrile illness caused by the protozoal organism of the genus Plasmodia. The vector for the transmission of the disease is the Anopheles mosquito [incorrect].

D. The Ixodes tick [incorrect], or the deer tick, is the vector for transmission of the treponemal organism, *Borrelia burgdoferi,* the causative organism of Lyme disease. This disorder begins with a characteristic skin rash (erythema chronicum migrans) with the development of musculoskeletal pains, cardiac and neurologic abnormalities, and finally severe arthritis.

E. The reduviid bug [correct], or kissing bug, is the vector for the causative organism of Chagas disease, caused by *Trypanosoma cruzi*. It is the leading cause of cardiac disease in some Latin American cultures, secondary to the resultant dilated cardiomyopathy that develops.

5-B

A. *Diphyllobothrium latum* [incorrect], also known as the fish tapeworm, is common in populations where raw or undercooked fish is eaten. The adult worm competes for vitamin B_{12}, causing megaloblastic anemia.

B. The causative agent of "river blindness" is *Onchocerca volvulus* [correct]. Transmitted by the black fly, the worms are not immunogenic until the microfilaria die, eliciting a significant immune response. Repeated cycles of damage lead to loss of vision.

C. *Ancylostoma duodenale* [incorrect], or hookworm, is a leading cause of iron deficiency anemias. The organism adheres to the intestinal mucosa, consuming 0.25 mL of blood/worm/day.

D. Visceral cutaneous migrans causes eosinophilia, pneumonitis, and hepatosplenomegaly. It is caused by the transmission of the ascaris nematode canis [incorrect] to humans via pets.

    E. African sleeping sickness, characterized by meningoencephalitis, is caused by the organism *Trypanosoma brucei* [incorrect]. This flaggelated protozoan is transmitted by the tsetse fly.

6-C

A. Cysticercosis results in the formation of fluid-filled cysts containing organisms within the brain. It results from the larval form of the pork tapeworm, *Taenia solium* [incorrect].

B. *Naegleria fowleri* [incorrect] is an ameba that can cause life-threatening meningoencephalitis. The organism is acquired by swimming in warm ponds and it gains access to the CNS via the cribriform plate.

C. Hydatid disease, characterized by the formation of cysts containing millions of scoleces, is a potentially lethal condition due to *Echinococcus granulosis* [correct].

D. *Trichinella spiralis* [incorrect] is acquired from the consumption of raw or undercooked pork. Larvae develop in skeletal muscle, resulting in persistent myalgias.

E. *Loa loa* [incorrect] is a filarial nematode also known as the African "eyeworm." The worms can be seen migrating beneath the conjunction in infected patients.

7-C

A. *Schistosoma mansoni*, a related trematode, inhabits the small branches of the inferior mesenteric vein. These trematode eggs, with sharp lateral spines, lodge in the portal tract, resulting in portal hypertension [incorrect].

B. Transitional cell carcinoma [incorrect] is the most common form of bladder cancer. Exposure to cigarette smoking and dyes used in the textile industry are frequently cited carcinogens.

C. The trematode *Schistosoma haematobium* migrates and resides in the urogenital tract, causing hematuria, dysuria, and urinary frequency. It is a recognized carcinogen for the development of squamous cell carcinoma of the bladder [correct].

D. Persistent *Helicobacter pylori* infection is associated with gastritis as well as gastric carcinoma. In addition, persistent infection is associated with monoclonal proliferation of B cells in the malt tissue of the GI tract, resulting in a maltoma [incorrect].

E. *Clonorchis sienesis* is a fluke (trematode) acquired by eating contaminated, undercooked fresh water fish. Infection by this organism, particularly prevalent in Asia, leads to chronic bile duct inflammation with the possibility of developing cholangiocarcinoma [incorrect].

8-D

A. Toxoplasmosis can be associated with exposure to contaminated feline feces. However it is not associated, as diseases like visceral larva migrans and echinococosis, with dog feces [incorrect].

B. Pinworm infection, caused by *Enterobius vermicularis*, and scabies are two common examples of diseases associated with direct person-to-person transmission [incorrect]. Such transmission often occurs under unsanitary conditions.

C. A common cause of diarrhea in AIDS patients is cryptosporidiosis. This organism is associated with consuming contaminated unchlorinated water [incorrect].

D. Consumption of raw meat [correct] is a common mode for Toxoplasmosis infection. It is one of the three major causes of a ring-enhancing mass on CT, along with brain abscesses and glioblastoma multiforme.

E. Cryptoccosis is an important cause of meningitis in patients with AIDS. It is often detected by India-ink staining of CSF. It is associated with exposure to contaminated pigeon droppings [incorrect].

9-A

A. Conjunctivitis due to adenovirus [correct] is commonly referred to as epidemic conjunctivitis. It is easily spread between infected individuals and from one eye to the other. Visual acuity is not affected without bacterial superinfection.

B. CMV [incorrect] can cause a severe, vision-threatening retinitis. However, it is rare in immunocompetent individuals.

C. HSV [incorrect] can cause a serious form of keratitis. It is the leading cause of corneal blindness in the United States.

D. Opthalmia neonatarum is a severe acute purulent conjunctivitis of the newborn. *Neisseria gonorrhea* [incorrect] is transferred to the delivered newborn by the mother. Patients are treated with silver nitrate eyedrops.

E. Trachomona, caused by *Chlamydia trachomatis* [incorrect] is the leading cause of blindness worldwide.

10-D

A. Elephantiasis, or lymphatic filariasis, results from infection by the roundworms *Wuchereria bancrofti* [incorrect] or *Brugia malayi*.

B. Rodents [incorrect] are the vector for numerous viral, as well as other, pathogens. Hantaan fever is a severe and potentially deadly disease transmitted by infected rodents.

C. The Culex mosquito [incorrect] can transmit filariasis as well as arboviruses such as the one that causes Japanese encephalitis.

D. Colorado tick fever is transmitted by the wood tick, Dermacentor [correct]. Other tick-borne illnesses include ehrlichiosis, Rocky Mountain spotted fever, and Lyme disease.

E. Bats [incorrect] are associated with two important illnesses. The bite of the bat can cause rabies and bat droppings, or guano, are associated with histoplasmosis.

11-C

A. Common unenveloped RNA viruses [incorrect] are rotavirus, picanovirus, and calcivirus. Although, these viruses are often, as a group, more likely to cause diarrheal illnesses.

B. A large majority of the medically relevant RNA viruses are enveloped [incorrect]. Two common enveloped RNA viruses that cause exanthems are rubella (a togavirus) and measles (a paramyxovirus).

C. This child presents with signs and symptoms of erythema infectiosum (fifth disease) that causes a rash, arthritis, and, in patients with hemolytic anemias, a transient aplastic crisis. This disorder results from infection with parvovirus B19—a single-stranded unenveloped DNA virus [correct].

D. Roseola infantum is another viral exanthem that also presents with a high fever. This condition is caused by HSV-6, a double-stranded enveloped DNA virus [incorrect].

E. The two medically important retroviruses [incorrect] are HIV and HTLV-1. Although each may be associated with dermatologic manifestations, neither presents as fifth disease.

12-A

A. Hepatitis A is an acute self-limiting illness due to a picornavirus. Usually transmitted via fecal/oral transmission, it almost always resolves without sequela [correct].

B. Fulminant hepatitis [incorrect] is a potentially life-threatening condition resulting from overwhelming liver damage. It is exceedingly rare in the case of viral infection and is much more common with exposure to drugs (halothane) or amanitin toxin (mushroom toxin).

C. There is no carrier state [incorrect] associated with HAV infection. However, patients infected with either HSV or HCV remain asymptomatic carriers of the respective virus.

D. Cirrhosis [incorrect] is a possibility in patients infected with both HBV and HCV, due to repeated episodes of hepatocellular scarring.

E. Hepatocellular carcinoma [incorrect] is again a possible consequence of either HBV or HCV infection. In the United States, HCV is more frequently associated with hepatocellular carcinoma.

13-B

A. The panel of diagnostic tests for choice A [incorrect] suggests that the patient has not been immunized appropriately to HBV. As well, he has not been infected with HBV. However, given his exposure, he is still at risk for transmission of other blood-borne pathogens (HIV-1, HCV, etc).

B. As choice B [correct] demonstrates, the patient does have antibodies to HBV surface antigen that are used in the preparation of the vaccine.

C. The patient with this profile [incorrect] does have a prior history of acute infection, which has since resolved.

D. This profile [incorrect] would be expected in a patient who has acute or chronic HBV infection.

E. The antibody profile for choice E [incorrect] would be expected for a patient with a later stage of a chronic infection.

14-D

A. Herpes Simplex Virus-I [incorrect] causes a painful vesicle lesion, most often on the lips or oral mucosa, whereas HSV-2 causes such lesions in the anogenital area. They can reactivate during times of stress or immunosupression.

B. CMV [incorrect] can cause hepatitis, colitis, and pneumonia; however, rarely does it have dermatologic manifestations in the adult.

C. Mononucleosis (EBV) [incorrect]. As it is transmitted by saliva, it is known to the public as the "kissing disease."

D. VZV [correct] is the herpes family member that causes both chicken pox as well as shingles (as in this case). Reactivation of the virus in times of suppressed immunity leads to a dermatomal distribution of vesicular lesions.

E. KSHV [incorrect] is the Karposi sarcoma–associated herpes virus. This virus causes a malignant tumor of the endothelial cells seen in AIDS patients as well as some Mediterranean populations.

15-E

A. DIC [incorrect] is a complication of the viruses that cause hemorrhagic fever, like Crimean-Congo virus, dengue fever virus, Marburg virus, and Ebola virus.

B. EBV is the cause of nasopharyngeal carcinoma [incorrect]. It is endemic to portions of Asia, especially Hong Kong.

C. Burkitt's lymphoma [incorrect], along with Hodgkin disease, is another EBV–virally associated neoplasm. Patients with endemic Burkitt–lymphoma in Africa manifest with jaw involvement, whereas sporadic cases, more common in the United States, involve the gastrointestinal tract.

D. Caused by a defective M protein of the measles virus, Subacute Sclerosing Panencephalitis [incorrect] a progressive fatal neurodegenerative condition.

E. Mumps can cause orchitis, which, when it occurs in a sexually mature individual, can cause sterility [correct] if bilateral testes are involved.

16-A

A. Rabies virus has a helical capsid, which is enveloped by electron microscopy, and it has a characteristic bullet shape [correct].

B. Flaviviruses, like the Ebola virus and the Marburg virus, have a distinctive filamentous [incorrect] virion.

C. Adenovirus particles are nonenveloped and icosahedral [correct]. The capsid is composed of 252 capsomeres with fibers projecting from each of the twelve verticies.

D. Poxviruses, the largest of the human viruses, have a destructive brick shape [incorrect].

E. *Yersenia pestis,* a bacteria, is often described as having the appearance of a safety pin [incorrect].

17-E

A. *Campylobacter jejuni* [incorrect] is a common cause of diarrhea in young children, often associated with contact with animals, e.g., puppies. However, the diarrhea is often bloody.

B. Rarely a problem in immunocompetent individuals, *Cryptosporidium parvum* [incorrect] is associated with chronic profuse, non bloody diarrhea. It is commonly a life-threatening condition in immunocompromised patients, like AIDS patients.

C. A common cause of epidemic dental illnesses, more commonly in adults is the Norwalk virus [incorrect]. This calcivirus is often the cause of diarrheal outbreaks on cruise ships.

D. Also known as the whipworm, the intestinal nematode *Trichuris trichiura* [incorrect] causes a chronic bloody diarrhea. Constant straining during prolonged bouts of diarrhea can lead to rectal prolapse.

E. The leading cause of diarrhea in children is rotavirus [correct]. This fecal locally transmitted virus causes an acute self-limiting diarrhea.

18-B

A. Prions are proteinaceous infectious particles that are neither viral nor bacterial. Cruetzfeld-Jakob disease is caused by a prion resulting in spongiform destruction of neurons with the development of myoclonus and invariably death.

B. SSPE results from a significant alteration in the matrix protein (M protein) [correct] of a measles virus. It is thought to be a late complication that results from a failure to completely clear a measles infection.

C. Congenital rubella [incorrect] causes a number of well-recognized defects in the neonate, including cataracts, microencephaly, congenital heart disease, and hepatosplenomegaly. Many of these defects are associated with several of the members of the TORCH group.

D. LCM Virus [incorrect] causes aseptic meningitis. It is contracted upon exposure to rodents and is found most commonly among laboratory workers and longshoremen.

E. Hepatitis D Virus [incorrect] is a defensive virus that requires coinfection with hepatitis B. Infection with these two viruses can lead to a potentially life-threatening fulminant hepatitis.

19-D

A. Rocky Mountain spotted fever (RMSF) is an acute, potentially fatal systemic vasculitis presenting with headache, fever, and rash. The causative organism of RMSF is the obligate intracellular organism, *Rickettsia rickettsii* [incorrect].

B. *Coxella burnetti* [incorrect] is the causative agent in Q fever. This condition manifests with headaches, fevers, and myalgias—it is associated most often with exposure to cattle, sheep, and goats.

C. *Rickettsia prowazekii* [incorrect] causes epidemic typhus. This louse-borne condition is associated with overcrowding and unsanitary conditions. The result is a serious systemic vasculitis complicated by encephalitis, myocarditis, pneumonia, and nephritis.

D. A cause of atypical pneumonia in humans in close contact with bird species of the psittaci group is *Chlamydia psittaci* [correct]. This is often an acute self-limiting illness in an era of antibiotics.

E. There are several serovars (immunologically distinct groups) of *Chlamydia trachomanis* [incorrect]. Serovars L1 and L2 are associated with lymphogranuloma venereum, whereas serovars A–C cause trachoma, a leading cause of blindness in the world.

20-D

A. One of the most common fungal pathogens is *Candida albicans*. Infection is often associated with immuno compromise, as in diabetes, AIDS, or chronic steroid use. Growth of these organisms in culture results in the formation of germ tubes [incorrect] at 37°C.

B. Broad-based budding [incorrect] describes the morphology of the dimorphic fungus, *Blastomyces dermatitidis*. This organism can cause suppurative granulomatous lesions in the lungs, skin, bones, and male genital tract.

C. Aspergillosis is one of the more common systemic mycoses, causing pulmonary symptoms as well as disseminated disease in immunocompromised individuals. The fungus that causes aspergillosis grows with septate hyphae branching at acute angles [incorrect] and can be seen in infected tissue.

D. Most often seen in diabetic individuals in ketoacidosis, mucormycosis is a potentially life-threatening cause of rhino-cerebral disease. The growth of this fungi is characterized by nonseptate hyphae that branch at >90° angles [correct].

E. Pityriasis versicolor is a common cause of skin rash due to the organism *Malassezia furfur*. The appearance of this organism is described as "spaghetti-and-meatballs" [incorrect] growth of tangled hyphae with clustered spherical budding yeast.

credits

Austen KF, Frank MM, Atkinson JP, et al. *Samter's Immunologic Diseases,* 6th ed. Philadelphia: Lippincott Williams & Wilkins; 2001. Fig. 44.4 (Case 65).

Barker LR, Fiebach NH, et al. *Principles of Ambulatory Medicine,* 7th ed. Philadelphia: Lippincott Williams & Wilkins; 2006. Figs. 109.4 (Case 54), 109.11 (Case 34).

Benjamin B, Hawke M, Stammberger H. *A Color Atlas of Otorinolaryngology.* Philadelphia: J.B. Lippincott Company; 1995. (Case 71).

Bhushan V, Le T, Pall V. *Underground Clinical Vignettes: Step One— Microbiology I,* 4th ed. Malden, Massachusetts: Blackwell Publishing; 2005. Figs. 016 (Case 17), 026 (Case 27), 028 (Case 29), 031 (Case 32), 036 (Case 37), 065 (Case 63), 073 (Case 70), 078 (Case 75), 084 (Case 80), 092 (Case 88).

Bhushan V, Le T, Pall V. *Underground Clinical Vignettes: Step One— Microbiology II,* 4th ed. Malden, Massachusetts: Blackwell Publishing; 2005. Fig. 027 (Case 95).

Corman ML. *Colon and Rectal Surgery,* 5th ed. Philadelphia: Lippincott Williams & Wilkins; 2004. Figs. 33-26 (Case 12), 33-21 (Case 16), 33-41 (Case 28), 20-5 (Case 51).

Crapo JD, Glassroth J, Karlinsky JB, et al. *Baum's Textbook of Pulmonary Disease,* 7th ed. Philadelphia: Lippincott Williams & Wilkins. Fig. 19.4 (Case 85 & 86).

Engleberg NC, Dermody T, DiRita V. *Schaechter's Mechanisms of Microbial Disease,* 4th ed. Philadelphia: Lippincott Williams & Wilkins; 2006. Figs. 43-4 (Case 48), 34-3 (Case 74), 34-1 (Case 74-2), (Case 35).

Engleberg NC, DiRita V, Dermody TS. *Schaechter's Mechanisms of Microbial Disease,* 4th ed. Philadelphia: Lippincott Williams & Wilkins; 2007: T33-1 (Case 79).

Fleisher GR, Ludwig S, Baskin MN. *Textbook of Pediatric Emergency Medicine*. Philadelphia: Lippincott Williams & Wilkins; 2004. Figs. 67.6 (Case 26), 94.12 A (Case 57), 84.28 (Case 100), T11.9 (Case 42).

Fu FH, Stone DA. *Sports Injuries: Mechanisms, Prevention and Treatment*, 2nd ed. Philadelphia: Lippincott Williams & Wilkins; 1994: T7.9 (Case 41). Fig. 47.6 (Case 91).

Goodheart HP. *Goodheart's Photoguide of Common Skin Disorders*, 2nd ed. Philadelphia: Lippincott Williams & Wilkins; 2003. Figs. 18.4 (Case 5), 17.3 (Case 8), 7.8 (Case 91).

Gorbach SL, Bartlett JG, Blacklow NR. *Infectious Diseases*, 3rd ed. Philadelphia: Lippincott Williams & Wilkins; 2003. Figs. 288.7A (Case 18), 288.6 (Case 18-2), 288.10 (Case 19), 286.3 (Case 22), 285.7 (Case 25), 143.1 (Case 43), 261.3 (Case 45), 139.10 (Case 53), 254.1 (Case 73), 139.9 (Case 78), 273.3 (Case 82), 272.2 (Case 90), 222.5 (Case 93).

Greenberg MJ, Hendrickson RG. *Greenberg's Text-Atlas of Emergency Medicine*. Philadelphia: Lippincott, Williams & Wilkins; 2004. Figs. 5-2 (Case 1), 20-20 (Case 20), 25-23 (Case 30), 33-8b (Case 31), 33-5 (Case 35), 5-32 (Case 50), 16-6 (Case 64), 5-19b (Courtesy of David Effron, MD) (Case 71), 20-35 (Case 87), 12-1 (Case 96), 12-6 (Case 97), T10-17B (Case 66).

Greer JP, Foerster J, Lukens JN, et al. *Wintrobe's Clinical Hematology*, 11th ed. Philadelphia: Lippincott Williams & Wilkins; 2003. Figs. 64.5 (Case 3), 94.13 (Case 58), 67.11.K (Case 59).

Hall JC. *Sauer's Manual of Skin Disorders*, 9th ed. Philadelphia: Lippincott Williams & Wilkins; 2006. Fig. 25-12A (Case 83).

Humes HD. *Kelley's Textbook of Internal Medicine*, 2nd ed. Philadelphia: Lippincott Williams & Wilkins; 2001. Figs. 324.1 (Case 11), 333.2 (Case 15), 308.3 (Case 44).

Kean BH, Sun T, Ellsworth RM. *Color atlas/text of ophthalmic parasitology*. New York: Igaku-Shoin; 1991. Fig. 121 (Case 24).

Knipe DM and Howley PM. *Field's Virology,* 5th ed. Philadelphia: Lippincott Williams & Wilkins; 2006. Figs. 6A & B – Ch 70 (Case 36), Fig. 6 – Ch 52 (Case 40), Fig. 10 – Ch 40 (Case 46).

Lee JK, Sagel SS, et al. *Computed Body Tomography with MRI Correlation,* 4th ed. Philadelphia: Lippincott Williams & Wilkins; 2005. Fig. 12-82 (Case 19).

McClatchey KD. *Clinical Laboratory Medicine,* 2nd ed. Philadelphia: Lippincott Williams & Wilkins; 2002. Figs. 60.29 (Case 17), 52.12 (Case 84) (Case 23).

McMillan JA, Fergin RD, et al. *Oski's Pediatrics: Principles and Practice,* 4th ed. Philadelphia: Lippincott Williams & Wilkins; 2006. Figs. 221.1 (Case 23), 77.4 (Case 38), 202.1 (Case 62), 197.1 (Case 72), 129.6 (Case 76), T431.2 (Case 7).

McClatchey KD, ed. *Clinical Laboratory Medicine,* 2nd ed. Philadelphia: Lippincott Williams & Wilkins; 2002: (Case 23).

Menkes JH, Sarnat HB, Maria BL. *Child Neurology,* 7th ed. Philadelphia: Lippincott Williams & Wilkins; 2005. Fig. 7.6 (Case 39), 7.9 (Case 68).

Oldham KT, Colombani PM, et al. *Principles and Practice of Pediatric Surgery.* Philadelphia: Lippincott Williams & Wilkins; 2004. Fig. 61-17 (Case 89).

Rowland LP. *Merritt's Neurology*, 11th ed. Philadelphia: Lippincott Williams & Wilkins; 2005. Fig. 24.7 (Case 69).

Rubin E, Gorstein F, Schwarting R, et al. *Rubin's Pathology: A Clinicopathologic Approach,* 4th ed. Baltimore: Lippincott Williams & Wilkins; 2004. Figs. 4-9 (Case 2), 9-86 (Case 21), 9-88 (Case 32), 9-89 (Case 33), 6-7 (Case 39), 9-6 (Case 52), 9-57 (Case 86), T4-2 (Case 6), T9-6 (Case 94).

Schiff ER, Sorrell MF, Maddrey WC. *Schiff's Diseases of the Liver,* 9th ed. Philadelphia: Lippincott Williams & Wilkins. Figs. 57.2 (Case 13), 4.40 (Case 49), 4.16 (Case 79).

Schwartz GR, Hanke BK, et al. *Principles and Practice of Emergency Medicine,* 4th ed. Philadelphia: Lippincott Williams & Wilkins. Fig. 61-4.3 (Case 42).

Smith C, Marks A, Lieberman M. Mark's Basic Medical Biochemistry: A Clinical Approach, 2nd ed. Philadelphia: Lippincott Williams & Wilkins; 2004. Fig. 24.12 (Case 4).

Tasman W, Jaeger E. *The Wills Eye Hospital Atlas of Clinical Ophthalmology*, 2nd ed. Lippincott Williams & Wilkins; 2001. Fig. 1.29 (Case 56).

case list

IMMUNOLOGY

1. Allergic Rhinitis
2. Anaphylaxis
3. Chédiak-Higashi Syndrome
4. Chronic Granulomatous Disease
5. Hereditary Angioedema
6. Selective Immunoglobulin A Deficiency
7. Severe Combined Immunodeficiency
8. Urticaria
9. Wiskott-Aldrich Syndrome
10. X-Linked Hypogammaglobulinemia

PARASITOLOGY

11. African Trypanosomiasis
12. Amebic Colitis
13. Amebic Liver Abscess
14. Amebic Meningoencephalitis
15. Anemia—*Diphyllobothrium Latum*
16. Chagas Disease
17. Cryptosporidiosis
18. Cysticercosis
19. Echinococcosis
20. Giardiasis
21. Hookworm Infection
22. Lymphatic Filariasis
23. Malaria
24. Onchocerciasis
25. Pinworm Infection
26. Scabies
27. Schistosomiasis
28. Urinary Schistosomiasis
29. Strongyloidiasis

30. Tick Paralysis
31. Toxoplasmosis
32. Trichinosis
33. Cutaneous Larva Migrans

VIROLOGY

34. Acute Conjunctivitis
35. Acquired Immunodeficiency Syndrome–Related Complex
36. Anemia—Aplastic Crisis (Parvovirus 19)
37. Cytomegalovirus Pneumonitis
38. Cytomegalovirus Retinitis
39. Cytomegalovirus—Congenital
40. Colorado Tick Fever
41. Common Cold (Viral)
42. Croup
43. Erythema Infectiosum
44. Hantaan Pulmonary Syndrome
45. Hemorrhagic Fever—Dengue
46. Hemorrhagic Fever—Ebola
47. Hepatitis A
48. Hepatitis B—Acute
49. Hepatitis C—Chronic Active
50. Herpangina
51. Herpes Genitalis
52. Herpes Simplex Encephalitis
53. Herpes Zoster (Shingles)
54. Herpes Zoster Ophthalmicus
55. Human Immunodeficiency Virus Transmission in Pregnancy
56. Herpes Simplex Virus Keratitis
57. Human Papillomavirus
58. Human T-Cell Leukemia Virus Type 1

59. Infectious Mononucleosis
60. Influenza
61. Lymphocytic Choriomeningitis
62. Measles
63. Molluscum Contagiosum
64. Mumps
65. Viral Myocarditis
66. Orchitis
67. Pericarditis
68. Poliomyelitis
69. Progressive Multifocal Leukoencephalopathy
70. Rabies
71. Ramsay-Hunt Syndrome
72. Roseola Infantum
73. Rotavirus Diarrhea
74. Respiratory Syncytial Virus Pneumonia
75. Rubella (German Measles)
76. Rubella—Congenital
77. Subacute Sclerosing Panencephalitis (SSPE)
78. Varicella (Chicken Pox)
79. Yellow Fever

MYCOLOGY

80. Aspergillosis
81. Aspergillosis—Allergic Bronchopulmonary
82. Blastomycosis
83. Candidiasis
84. Coccidioidomycosis
85. Histoplasmosis
86. Meningitis—Cryptococcal
87. Mucormycosis
88. Pityriasis Versicolor
89. *Pneumocystis Carinii* Pneumonia
90. Sporotrichosis
91. Tinea Cruris (Ringworm/Jock Itch)

RICKETTSIA AND CHLAMYDIA

92. *Chlamydia* Pneumonia
93. *Chlamydia Trachomatis*
94. Endemic Typhus
95. Epidemic Typhus
96. Epididymitis
97. Lymphogranuloma Venereum
98. Psittacosis
99. Q Fever
100. Rocky Mountain Spotted Fever

index

Abdominal abscess, 24
ABPA. *See* Allergic bronchopul-
  monary aspergillosis
Actinomycosis, 164, 174
Acute conjunctivitis, 67–68
Acute respiratory distress
  syndrome, 87–88, 178
African trypanosomiasis,
  21–22, 46, 211
Agammaglobulinemia, 18
AIDS/HIV, 22, 61, 75, 78, 94,
  105, 116, 118, 160, 166,
  171, 210
  cryptosporidiosis and, 33–34
  molluscum contagiosum
    and, 125–126
  PCP and, 177–178
  PML and, 137–138
  transmission in pregnancy,
    109–110
AIDS-related complex (ARC),
  69–70
Albinism, 5–6
Alcoholic hepatitis, 96
Allergic bronchopulmonary
  aspergillosis (ABPA),
  161–162
Allergic rhinitis, 1–2
Amebiasis, 34
Amebic colitis, 23–24
Amebic hepatic abscess, 38
Amebic liver abscess, 25–26
Amebic meningoencephalitis,
  27–28, 122
Amyloidosis, 56, 130

Anaphylaxis, 3–4, 10
Anemia
  aplastic, 20
  aplastic crisis (parvovirus
    19), 71–72
  Diphyllobothrium latum,
    29–30
  iron deficiency, 42
  pernicious, 30
  sickle cell, 71
Angioedema, 4, 9–10, 64
Anthrax, 188, 190
Aplastic anemia, 20
ARC. *See* AIDS-related complex
Atrioventricular malformation,
  24
Aseptic meningitis, 28, 104,
  136, 172
Aspergillosis, 159–160, 164,
  170, 218. *See also* Allergic
  bronchopulmonary
  aspergillosis
Aspiration, 2
Asthma, 10, 58, 148, 160, 162
Atopic dermatitis, 18, 106,
  126, 166
Autoimmune hepatitis, 96, 98

Babesia microti infection, 22
Babesiosis, 168
Bacillary angiomatosis, 70
Bacterial gastroenteritis, 42, 146
Bacterial meningitis, 28, 122,
  172
Bacterial parotitis, 128

Bacterial pharyngitis, 100
Bacterial pneumonia, 74, 196
Basal cell carcinoma, 126
B-cell disorder, 12, 14, 18
Bell palsy, 60, 142
Bilharziasis. See Schistosomiasis
Biliary disease, 26, 38
Bioterrorism, 88
Bladder cancer, 56
Blastomycosis, 163–164, 170, 180
Botulism, 60, 136
Brain abscess, 36, 62, 154
Bronchiectasis, 162
Bronchiolitis, 148
Bronchitis, 2, 82
Brucelliosis, 22
Bruton agammaglobulinemia, 8, 18, 20
Budd-Chiari syndrome, 38, 94
Bullous pemphigoid, 16
Burkitt lymphoma, 118, 205, 216

Calabar edema, 48
Calculus of Stensen duct, 128
Campylobacter infection, 34
Cancer
  bladder, 56
  cervical, 114
  esophageal, 32
  urethral, 54
Candidiasis, 13, 50, 165–166, 182
Celiac sprue, 40
Cellulitis, 174
Cercarial dermatitis, 55
Cervical cancer, 114
Chagas disease, 31–32, 130, 211

Chancroid, 102
Chédiak-Higashi syndrome, 5–6
Chicken pox, 52, 102, 126, 155–156. See also Varicella-zoster virus
Chlamydia pneumonia, 170, 183–184, 196
Chlamydia trachomatis, 185–186, 203, 207, 217
Cholangitis, 98
Cholera, 146
Chronic bronchitis, 2
Chronic fatigue syndrome, 198
Chronic granulomatous disease, 6, 7–8, 20, 209
Chronic lymphocytic leukemia (CLL), 119
Chronic pruritus, 16
CLL. See Chronic lymphocytic leukemia
CMV. See Cytomegalovirus
CNS neoplasm, 36
Coccidioidomycosis, 167–168
Colitis, 23–24
Collagen vascular disease, 72
Colorado tick fever, 79–80, 213
Combined B-cell and T-cell disorders, 12
Common cold (viral), 81–82
Common variable immunodeficiency, 8
Complex partial seizure, 104
Condyloma acuminatum, 126
Congestive heart failure, 88
Conjunctivitis, 67–68, 108, 188, 213
Contact dermatitis, 52, 102, 106, 150, 156

Corneal abrasion, 68
Coxsackie virus infection, 82, 99–100, 130, 134
Creutzfeldt-Jakob disease, 140
Crimean Congo fever, 90, 92
Crohn disease, 40
Croup, 83–84, 148
Cryptococcosis, 164, 213
Cryptosporidiosis, 33–34, 216
Cryptosporidium infection, 40
Cutaneous larva migrans, 65–66
Cutaneous T-cell lymphoma, 6
Cystic fibrosis, 20
Cysticercosis, 35–36, 38, 211
Cytomegalovirus (CMV), 94, 201, 203, 205, 210, 213, 215
  congenital, 77–78
  infection, 34, 70
  infectious mononucleosis and, 118
  PCP and, 178
  pneumonitis, 73–74
  retinitis, 75–76

Dengue fever, 46, 89–90, 92, 158
Dermatitis herpetiformis, 16
Diabetes, 70
DiGeorge syndrome, 18, 152, 201
Diphtheria, 84
Diphyllobothrium latum, 29–30
Disseminated gonococcal disease, 200
Diverticulitis, 58
Diverticulosis, 24
Dressler syndrome, 130

Ebola virus, 90, 91–92
EBV. *See* Epstein-Barr virus
Echinococcosis, 28, 37–38, 212
Echinococcosis hydatid cyst, 26
Eczema, 17–18, 50
Ehrlichiosis, 80, 188, 190
Emphysema, 2
Encephalitis, 36, 172
Endemic typhus, 187–188, 190
Endocardial fibroelastosis, 130
Enteroviral infection, 76, 78, 100
Eosinophilia, 47, 53, 57–58, 63, 160
  hookworm infection and, 42
  lymphatic filariasis and, 43
Epidemic typhus, 188, 189–190
Epididymitis, 132, 191–192
Epiglottitis, 10, 84
Epstein-Barr virus (EBV), 94, 205
Erythema infectiosum, 85–86, 144
Esophageal cancer, 32
Esophageal rupture, 134
Esophagitis, 134

Folliculitis, 52
Food poisoning, 64
Foreign body aspiration, 2
Fungal pneumonia, 74

Gastritis, 134
Gastroenteritis, 42, 64, 146
Gastroesophageal reflux disease, 32, 162
German measles. *See* Rubella
Giardiasis, 34, 39–40

Glaucoma, 68, 108
Guillain-Barré syndrome, 136, 140

Hand, foot, and mouth disease (HFMD), 86, 100, 200
Hantaan pulmonary syndrome, 87–88
Hemochromatosis, 96, 98
Hemorrhagic cystitis, 56
Hemorrhagic fever—Dengue. See Dengue fever
Hemorrhagic fever—Ebola. See Ebola virus
Hepatitis
  alcoholic, 96
  autoimmune, 96
Hepatitis A, 93–94, 96, 201
Hepatitis B
  acute, 95–96
  chronic, 98
Hepatitis C—chronic active, 97–98
Hepatocellular carcinoma, 26
Hereditary angioedema, 9–10
Hernia, 132
Herpangina, 99–100
Herpes genitalis, 101–102
Herpes simplex, 100, 106, 203, 205, 215
  chicken pox and, 156
  molluscum contagiosum and, 126
Herpes simplex encephalitis, 103–104, 122
Herpes simplex keratitis, 111–112
Herpes zoster, 60, 76, 78, 102, 105–106
  acute conjunctivitis and, 68

Ramsay-Hunt syndrome and, 142
Herpes zoster ophthalmicus, 107–108
HFMD. See hand, foot, and mouth disease
Hidradenitis, 114
Histoplasmosis, 169–170
HIV. See AIDS/HIV
HIV wasting syndrome, 34
Hodgkin disease, 194
Hookworm infection, 41–42
HPV. See Human papillomavirus
HTLV-1. See Human T-cell leukemia virus type 1
Human immunodeficiency virus infection, 8, 13–14
Human papillomavirus (HPV), 113–114
Human T-cell leukemia virus type 1 (HTLV-1), 115–116, 214
Hydatid cyst, 26
Hydatid disease. See Echinococcosis
Hydrocele, 132, 192
Hyperimmunoglobulinemia E syndrome, 8, 13–14
Hypersensitivity pneumonitis, 66
Hypersensitivity reactions, 4, 13, 48, 130
Hypersensitivity vasculitis, 16
Hypertrophic cardiomyopathy, 32
Hypogammaglobulinemia, 20

IDDM. See Insulin-dependent diabetes mellitus

IgA deficiency, 11–12, 209
IgE-mediated type I
    hypersensitivity reaction, 4
Immunodeficiency, 8, 12,
    13–14
Impetigo, 106, 156, 182
Infectious mononucleosis, 20,
    117–118, 120, 215
  malaria and, 46
  rubella and, 150
Inflammatory bowel disease, 58
Inflammatory proctocolitis, 194
Influenza, 64, 74, 82,
    118–120, 148, 184, 198
Insulin-dependent diabetes
    mellitus (IDDM), 173
Intracranial abscess, 104
Iritises, 68
Iron deficiency anemia, 42
Irritable bowel syndrome, 40
Isosporiasis, 34

Job syndrome, 8, 13–14
Jock itch. *See* Tinea cruris

Kawasaki disease, 124
Keratitis, 108, 111–112
Keratoconjunctitis sicca, 112
Korean hemorrhagic fever, 88

Laryngeal edema, 10
LCM. *See* Lymphocytic
    choriomeningitis
Legionnaire disease, 184, 196
Leishmaniasis, 32, 54, 180
Leprosy, 44, 48
Leptomeningeal carcinomatosis,
    104
Leptospirosis, 46, 90, 154,
    188, 190

Leukocyte adhesion deficiency, 8
Lice, 52
Lichen planus, 50
Löffler syndrome, 66, 162
Löffler pneumonitis, 42
Ludwig angina, 10
Lyme disease, 80, 130, 200
Lymphatic filariasis, 43–44
Lymphedema, 44
Lymphocytic choriomeningitis
    (LCM), 76, 78, 121–122,
    206
Lymphogranuloma venereum,
    193–194
Lymphohistiocytosis, 13–14
Lymphoma, 20, 44, 62, 170
Lymphoproliferative disorders,
    13–14
Lymphosarcoma, 44

Malaria, 22, 32, 45–46, 54, 90,
    211
  amebic liver abscess and,
    26
  amebic meningoencephalitis
    and, 28
Malignant carcinoid syndrome, 4
Marburg virus, 92
Measles, 123–124, 144, 154,
    200, 206
  erythema infectiosum and, 86
  rubella and, 150
Medullary carcinoma of
    thyroid, 4
Meningeal carcinomatosis,
    172
Meningitis, 36, 154, 198
  aseptic, 28, 104, 136, 172
  bacterial, 28, 122, 172
  cryptococcal, 171–172

Meningococcemia, 144
Meningoencephalitis, 27–28
Migraine headache, 104
Mikulicz syndrome, 128
Mixed connective-tissue
    disease, 2
Molluscum contagiosum, 114,
    125–126
Mononucleosis. *See* Infectious
    mononucleosis
Mucormycosis, 173–174
Multiple sclerosis, 60, 138
Mumps, 86, 118, 127–128,
    132, 216
Myeloproliferative disease, 54
Myocardial infarction, 134
Myocarditis, 129–130

Neuroblastoma, 152
Nocardiosis, 174
Non-Hodgkin lymphoma, 105,
    116, 194

Onchocerciasis, 47–48, 211
Orchitis, 131–132
Otitis media, 19

Paracoccidioidomycosis, 180
Parainfluenza, 82, 120
Parotitis, 127–128
Parvovirus 19, 71–72, 124, 150
Patent ductus arteriosus (PDA),
    151
PCP. *See Pneumocystis carinii*
    pneumonia
PDA. *See* Patent ductus
    arteriosus
Pericarditis, 133–134
Peritonsillar abscess, 10
Pernicious anemia, 30

Pharyngitis, 100, 118
Pheochromocytoma, 4
Pinworm infection, 49–50, 212
Pityriasis alba, 176
Pityriasis versicolor, 175–176,
    218
Plummer-Vinson syndrome, 42
PML. *See* Progressive multifocal
    leukoencephalopathy
Pneumocystis carinii pneumonia
    (PCP), 177–178
Pneumonia, 11, 88, 120,
    147–148, 160, 178, 198
    bacterial, 74, 196
    Chlamydia, 74
    fungal, 74
Pneumonic plague, 88
Poliomyelitis, 135–136, 140
Polyarteritis nodosa, 64
Proctitis, 50
Progressive multifocal
    leukoencephalopathy
    (PML), 137–138
Pruritic urticarial papules and
    plaques of pregnancy
    (PUPPP), 16
Pruritus, 16
Psittacosis, 184, 195–196
Psoriasis, 52, 182
PUPPP. *See* Pruritic urticarial
    papules and plaques of
    pregnancy
Pyoderma gangrenosum, 6

Q fever, 80, 184, 196, 197–198

Rabies, 28, 136, 139–140, 216
Ramsay-Hunt syndrome,
    141–142
Reiter syndrome, 188

Respiratory syncytial virus (RSV)
    infection, 82
    pneumonia, 147–148
Retropharyngeal abscess, 84
Rheumatic heart disease, 130
Ringworm. *See* Tinea cruris
River blindness. *See*
    Onchocerciasis
RMSF. *See* Rocky Mountain
    spotted fever
Rocky Mountain spotted fever
    (RMSF), 199–200, 210,
    217
    Colorado tick fever and, 80
    typhus and, 188, 190
Romaña sign, 31
Rose gardener's disease. *See*
    Sporotrichosis
Roseola infantum, 86,
    143–144, 214
Rotavirus diarrhea, 145–146
RSV. *See* Respiratory syncytial
    virus
Rubella, 72, 76, 78, 118, 124,
    144, 149–150, 206, 214
    congenital, 151–152, 217
Rubeola. *See* Measles

Salmonella, 146
Salmonellosis, 34
Sarcoidosis, 62, 130, 168, 170
Scabies, 51–52, 212
Scalded skin syndrome, 124
Scarlet fever, 72, 86, 118
Schistosomiasis, 38, 53–54
    urinary, 55–56
SCID. *See* Severe combined
    immunodeficiency
Scleritis, 68, 108
Seborrheic dermatitis, 176

Selective IgA deficiency, 11–12
Severe combined
    immunodeficiency (SCID),
    12, 13–14, 201, 210
    Wiskott-Aldrich syndrome
    and, 18
    X-linked hypogammaglobu-
    linemia and, 20
Shigellosis, 24
Shingles. *See* Herpes zoster
Short-gut syndrome, 30
Sicca syndrome, 188
Sickle-cell anemia, 71
Sinusitis, 2, 11
Slapped-cheek appearance, 85
Sleeping sickness. *See* African
    trypanosomiasis
Smallpox, 106, 156
Sporotrichosis, 44, 179–180
SSPE. *See* Subacute sclerosing
    panencephalitis
Staphylococcal infection, 166,
    168, 180
Steeple sign, 83
Streptococcal infection, 166
Strongyloidiasis, 57–58
Subacute sclerosing
    panencephalitis (SSPE),
    124, 153–154, 205, 217
Swimmer's itch, 53
Syphilis, 48, 102, 116, 200
Systemic mastocytosis, 4

Taenia infection, 30
T-cell disorder, 12, 14, 18
Temporomandibular joint
    syndrome, 142
Testicular torsion, 132, 192
Testicular tumor, 132
Tetanus, 136, 140

Thrombocytopenia, 18
Tick paralysis, 59–60
Tinea corporis, 176
Tinea cruris, 50, 181–182
Tinea infection, 66
Tinea versicolor, 182
Toxoplasmosis, 32, 61–62, 78,
    138, 152, 172, 212
    amebic meningoencephalitis
        and, 28
    CMV retinitis and, 76
    SSPE and, 154
Tracheitis, 84
Trichinosis, 63–64
Trigeminal neuralgia, 108
Trisomy, 152
Tuberculoma, 36
Tuberculosis, 22, 28, 62, 154,
    164, 178, 184
    ARC and, 70
    aspergillosis and, 160
    urinary schistosomiasis and,
        56
Tularemia, 80, 180, 188, 190,
    196
Typhoid fever, 26, 54, 64, 90, 92
Typhus, 187–188, 189–190

Urethral cancer, 54
Urinary schistosomiasis,
    55–56
Urticaria, 15–16, 52, 66, 156
Uveitis, 68, 188

Varicella-zoster virus (VZV),
    74, 106, 108, 205, 215
Vasculitis, 66
Viral myocarditis, 129–130
Viral parotitis, 128
Vitamin A deficiency, 48
Vitiligo, 176
VZV. See Varicella-zoster virus

Wegener granulomatosis, 160,
    162
West Nile virus, 90, 122
Wilson disease, 96, 98
Wiskott-Aldrich syndrome, 12,
    13–14, 17–18, 20, 201,
    209

X-linked hypogammaglobuline-
    mia, 20

Yellow fever, 90, 92, 157–158